Peter Voitl

Physiologic effects of rotary blood pumps

Peter Voitl

Physiologic effects of rotary blood pumps

Physiologische Auswirkungen von Rotationspumpen

Südwestdeutscher Verlag für Hochschulschriften

Impressum/Imprint (nur für Deutschland/ only for Germany)
Bibliografische Information der Deutschen Nationalbibliothek: Die Deutsche Nationalbibliothek verzeichnet diese Publikation in der Deutschen Nationalbibliografie; detaillierte bibliografische Daten sind im Internet über http://dnb.d-nb.de abrufbar.
Alle in diesem Buch genannten Marken und Produktnamen unterliegen warenzeichen-, markenoder patentrechtlichem Schutz bzw. sind Warenzeichen oder eingetragene Warenzeichen der jeweiligen Inhaber. Die Wiedergabe von Marken, Produktnamen, Gebrauchsnamen, Handelsnamen, Warenbezeichnungen u.s.w. in diesem Werk berechtigt auch ohne besondere Kennzeichnung nicht zu der Annahme, dass solche Namen im Sinne der Warenzeichen- und Markenschutzgesetzgebung als frei zu betrachten wären und daher von jedermann benutzt werden dürften.

Verlag: Südwestdeutscher Verlag für Hochschulschriften Aktiengesellschaft & Co. KG
Dudweiler Landstr. 99, 66123 Saarbrücken, Deutschland
Telefon +49 681 37 20 271-1, Telefax +49 681 37 20 271-0, Email: info@svh-verlag.de
Zugl.: Wien, Medizinische Universität, Dissertation, 2008

Herstellung in Deutschland:
Schaltungsdienst Lange o.H.G., Berlin
Books on Demand GmbH, Norderstedt
Reha GmbH, Saarbrücken
Amazon Distribution GmbH, Leipzig
ISBN: 978-3-8381-0766-0

Imprint (only for USA, GB)
Bibliographic information published by the Deutsche Nationalbibliothek: The Deutsche Nationalbibliothek lists this publication in the Deutsche Nationalbibliografie; detailed bibliographic data are available in the Internet at http://dnb.d-nb.de.
Any brand names and product names mentioned in this book are subject to trademark, brand or patent protection and are trademarks or registered trademarks of their respective holders. The use of brand names, product names, common names, trade names, product descriptions etc. even without a particular marking in this works is in no way to be construed to mean that such names may be regarded as unrestricted in respect of trademark and brand protection legislation and could thus be used by anyone.

Publisher:
Südwestdeutscher Verlag für Hochschulschriften Aktiengesellschaft & Co. KG
Dudweiler Landstr. 99, 66123 Saarbrücken, Germany
Phone +49 681 37 20 271-1, Fax +49 681 37 20 271-0, Email: info@svh-verlag.de

Copyright © 2009 by the author and Südwestdeutscher Verlag für Hochschulschriften Aktiengesellschaft & Co. KG and licensors
All rights reserved. Saarbrücken 2009

Printed in the U.S.A.
Printed in the U.K. by (see last page)
ISBN: 978-3-8381-0766-0

Table of Content

English Abstract	4
Deutsches Abstract	6
1. Introduction	9
1.1 Cardiac Insufficiency	9
1.1.1 Prevention	13
1.1.2 Prognosis	16
1.1.3 Therapy	18
1.2 Types of support	22
1.2.1 Pulsatile Systems	24
1.2.2 Continous flow systems	26
1.3 Clinical used rotary pump systems	28
1.3.1 The DuraHeart System	30
1.3.2 The Berlin Heart	31
1.3.3 The HeartMate II	32
1.3.4 The MicroMed DeBakey VAD	33
1.3.5 The HeartWare LVAD	34
1.3.6 VentrAssist LVAD	35
1.4 Indications	36
1.4.1 Rescue support	36
1.4.2 Bridge to heart transplant	36
1.4.3 Bridge to myocardial recovery	38
1.4.4 Permanent assist device	39
1.5 Contraindications	41
1.6 Complications	42
1.7 Trends and developments	45

2. Physiology of Reduced Pulsatility   46

    2.1 Effects on the circulation   48
    2.2 Effects on cerebral function
        and the nervous system   52
    2.3 Effects on splanchnic organ function
        and kidney function   53
    2.4 Effects on pulmonary function   55
    2.5 Effects on endocrine function   56
    2.6 Outcome   57

3. Own Results   60

    3.1   Coronary hemodynamics and
          myocardial oxygen consumption during
          support with rotary blood pumps   60
          3.1.1 Abstract   61
          3.1.2 Introduction   62
          3.1.3 Methods   63
          3.1.4 Results   64
          3.1.5 Discussion   66
          3.1.6 Conclusion   68

    3.2   Suction events during left ventricular support and
          ventricular arrhythmias   69
          3.2.1 Abstract   70
          3.2.2 Introduction   71
          3.2.3 Methods   72
          3.2.4 Results   76
          3.2.5 Discussion   84
          3.2.6 Conclusion   86

4. Conclusion   87

5. References   88

Für Regine.

English Abstract

The use of rotary blood pumps for assistance of advanced heart failure continues to increase with the growing prevalence of the disease itself and the availability of small and clinically applicable devices. These devices are used either as cardiac support prior to transplantation or to assist the recovery of the heart. As rotary blood pumps produce a non-pulsatile flow, several questions concerning the physiology of pulseless circulation are remaining. The first part of this thesis gives an introduction on cardiac support with blood pumps and covers the physiology of low-pulse and pulseless circulation under rotary assist device support according to the literature.

The second part is presenting own scientific work on the topic of the thesis. Two publications resulted from the scientific focus, the first project deals with the effects of left ventricular assist device therapy on coronary hemodynamics, myocardial oxygen consumption and pulmonary blood flow in sheep. An in vivo investigation in 10 sheep was done to determine invasively measured coronary perfusion data as well as pressure and flow conditions under cardiovascular assistance and compare the effects of the assistance to physiologic circulatory conditions.

A DeBakey VAD® was implanted and systemic and coronary hemodynamic measurements were performed at defined baseline conditions where up to five levels of assistance were tested. Our results reflect that blood flow in the coronary arteries does not correlate with changes in pump flow of rotary blood pumps. The changes in the pulmonary artery could reflect a drop in pulmonary vascular resistance: an effect that eventually may contribute in significant measure to the stabilization of the right ventricle. A change in the geometry of the left ventricle due to the unloading may be an alternative explanation. Particularly this unaltered coronary perfusion at falling oxygen consumption might contribute to cardiac recovery.

The second project refers to endocardial suction that can occur with rotary pumps as well as with pulsatile pumps, leading to possible ventricular collapse, suction of the ventricular wall and subsequent right ventricular dysfunction. We report severe ventricular arrhythmias closely related to suction events in rotary blood pumps, a phenomenon that has not been described before.

Our aim was to find arrhythmias related to suction and classify them either as monomorphic ventricular tachycardia (single beat), monomorphic ventricular tachycardia (series) or as polymorphic ventricular tachycardia. 19 patients underwent an overall number of 57 measurement sessions. The electrocardiagramms were classified semi-manually aided be a graphical user interface. It was observed that excessive ventricular unloading of the left ventricle during continuous left ventricular support can induce ventricular arrhythmias; there is also an evidence for an increase of arrhythmic activity after suction. This turned out to be a transient effect, which vanishes within five minutes after suction. The ECG-events related to suction have a sudden onset and are severe ventricular arrhythmias, which can consist of even just one extrasystolic beat and they usually cease after clearance of suction. We conclude that suction events in rotary blood pumps can cause severe ventricular arrhythmias and need to be avoided. Whether these post-LVAD ventricular arrhythmias are associated with an adverse outcome needs to be investigated further.

Deutsches Abstract

Die Verwendung axialer Blutpumpen zur Unterstützung des Herzens bei fortgeschrittenem Herzversagen nimmt zu, einerseits aufgrund der steigenden Prävalenz von Herz- und Kreislauferkrankungen, andererseits aufgrund der Verfügbarkeit von kleinen und klinisch anwendbaren axialen Pumpen. Diese Systeme finden entweder Verwendung als Herzunterstützung im Rahmen der Überbrückung und Vorbereitung auf eine Herztransplantation; andererseits um die Erholung des Herzens zu unterstützen. Axiale Blutpumpen zeichnen sich durch einen niedrig pulsatilen oder sogar non-pulsatilen Blutfluss aus, was zahlreiche Fragen zur Physiologie aufwirft.

Im ersten Teil dieser Dissertation wird ein Überblick über die Herzkreislaufunterstützung mittels Kunstherzen gegeben und anhand der aktuellen Literatur die Physiologie eines Kreislaufs mit herabgesetzter oder fehlender Pulsatilität beschrieben. Im zweiten Teil werden eigene wissenschaftliche Arbeiten zum Thema präsentiert.

Das erste Projekt behandelt den Effekt einer axialen Blutpumpe auf die koronare Durchblutung, den myocardialen Sauerstoffverbrauch und den pulmonalen Blutfluss bei Schafen. Eine in vivo Untersuchung wurde an 10 Schafen durchgeführt, um koronare Durchblutungsparameter wie auch die Druck- und Blutflussverhältnisse sowohl mit als auch ohne Unterstützung mit axialen Blutpumpen invasiv zu messen und zu vergleichen.

Ein DeBakey VAD wurde implantiert und die systemischen und koronaren Blutflüsse sowohl unter baseline Bedingungen als auch unter unterschiedlichen Levels der Pumpeneinstellungen gemessen. Unsere Resultate weisen darauf hin, dass der Blutfluss der Koronararterien nicht mit den Veränderungen an den Einstellungen der Pumpe korreliert. Die Veränderungen des pulmonalen Blutflusses können auf einen herabgesetzten pulmonalen Gefäßwiderstand hindeuten; ein Effekt der zu einer Stabilisierung des rechten Ventrikels beitragen könnte;

möglicherweise auch aufgrund einer Veränderung der Geometrie des linken Ventrikels durch die Volumsentlastung. Gerade diese gleich bleibende koronare Durchblutung bei sinkendem Sauerstoffverbrauch des Myocards kann zur Herzerholung beitragen.

Das zweite Projekt befasst sich mit Ansaugereignissen im linken Ventrikel, die während dieser Form der Herzunterstützung gleichermaßen wie bei einer Unterstützung mit pulsatilen Kunstherzen auftreten können. Endokardiales Ansaugen kann zu einem möglichen linksventrikulärem Kollaps, Ansaugen der Wand des Ventrikels und nachfolgender rechtsventrikulärer Dysfunktion führen. Ziel dieses Teils der Dissertation war es, schwere ventrikuläre Arrhythmien darzustellen und zu klassifizieren, die in einem zeitlichen Bezug zu Ansaugereignissen stehen.

Das Ziel war es, ventrikuläre Arrhythmien in einem zeitlichen Zusammenhang mit Ansaugereignissen darzustellen und diese morphologisch zu klassifizieren. Als Einteilung wurde die monomorphe ventriculäre Tachycardie (Einzelschlag) von der monomorphen ventriculären Tachycardie (als Serie) und von der polymorphen ventriculären Tachycardie abgegrenzt. 19 Patienten wurden einer Gesamtzahl von 57 Untersuchungen unterzogen. Die Elektrokardiogramme wurden semi-manuell mittels eines graphischen Interface in der Software Matlab klassifiziert.

Es zeigte sich, dass die exzessive Entleerung des linken Ventrikels während des Supports ventrikuläre Arrhythmien induzieren kann; es gibt Hinweise für einen Anstieg von arrhythmischen Ereignissen nach dem Ansaugen. Dabei handelt es sich um einen transienten Effekt, der 5 Minuten nach dem Suction-Ereignis nicht mehr nachweisbar ist. Diese EKG Veränderungen haben einen plötzlichen Beginn und sind schwerwiegende ventrikuläre Ereignisse, die in aller Regel nach Ende des Ansaugens verschwinden. Wenngleich weiterführende Untersuchungen notwendig sind, um festzustellen inwieweit diese Arrhythmien mit einem schlechteren Outcome korrelieren, weisen diese Daten darauf hin, dass Ansaugereignisse vermieden werden sollen.

Zahlreiche rezente Studien haben das exzellente Potential axialer Herzpumpen gezeigt, um Patienten mit terminalem Herzversagen mit einer guten Lebensqualität unterstützen zu können. Die Effekte eines niedrig pulsatilen Kreislaufs oder einer überhaupt pulslosen Zirkulation auf die Physiologie sind noch nicht vollständig bekannt. Diese Daten sollen dazu beitragen, zukünftige Rotationspumpensysteme weiter zu verbessern.

1 Introduction

Currently the main indication for artificial blood pumps is terminal cardiac insufficiency without any perspective for improvement by conventional medical therapy. The mechanical support of the heart and the cardiovascular system is established as a bridging therapy to heart transplantation as well as part of a concept for treatment of patients with terminal cardiac insufficiency who are not eligible for transplantation and remain in a state of cardiac decompensation after appropriate medical therapy.

These systems are usually implanted as bridge to transplant, as bridge to recovery as alternative to transplant or as rescue support. Artificial blood pump support of the heart offers the possibility of fast stabilisation and mobilization of the patients. All the currently used systems are rather expensive and should remain in the responsibility of specialised transplant centres based on the current state of the art [1-3]. From the physiologic point of view it is important to distinguish two different types of devices by the produced flow pattern, which may be either a pulsatile or a continous flow.

1.1 Cardiac Insufficiency

Cardiac insufficiency is an important reason for hospital admissions.

The wide range of definitions used in clinical trials makes it difficult to interpret the published data in determining the incidence of heart failure in cardiovascular studies and the effects of interventions on these endpoints[4].

In Germany as in other industrialised countries it is one of the leading causes of mortality, morbidity and disability. The direct costs of heart failure in 2004 in Germany were 2,548 Million Euro. Especially hospitalisation related to progression of the disease is a problem [5].

The Rotterdam study states that in individuals aged 55, almost 1 in 3 will develop heart failure during their remaining lifespan [6].

In the USA about 400.000 patients with cardiac insufficiency have been registered in 1991[7], in 2006 a heart failure incidence of 19.3 per 1000 person years has been published[8]; the rate of first hospitalized myocardial insufficiency or coronary heart disease death was 19.2 events per 1000 person years. Heart failure continues to be a fatal disease, with only 35% surviving 5 years after the first diagnosis[6].

It is a multifactorial disease and thus is being influenced by a variety of different risk factors such as environmental and genetic and it is difficult to identify the most relevant risk factors involved in the individual development of the disease. The reasons include coronary artery disease, congenital heart disease, valvular heart disease, cardiomyopathy and patients after heart transplant with coronary heart disease and cardiomyopathy as the leading factors.

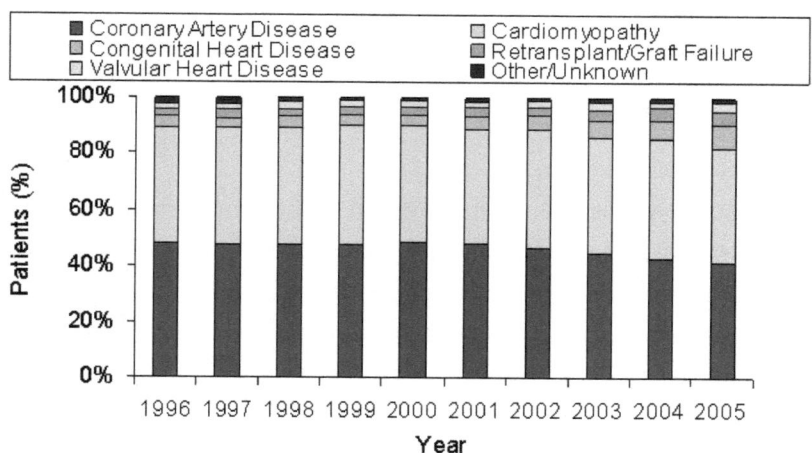

Fig 1: Diagnosis related to severe cardiac insufficiency
Annual Report of the U.S. Organ Procurement and Transplantation Network OPTH/SRTR 2006, Table 11.1a

		2002	2003	2004	2005	2006	2005/ 2006
Heart	heart	418	556	713	864	904	4.6%
	heart + liver	1	0	0	0	1	0.0%
	heart + liver + lung	1	0	0	0	0	0.0%
	heart + lung	42	45	54	64	59	-7.8%
	kidney + heart	4	12	15	18	15	-16.7%
Heart	total	466	613	782	946	979	3.5%

Fig 2: Active Eurotransplant waiting list
Annual Report 2006 of the Eurotransplant Foundation[3]

The Eurotransplant Foundation reports an increase in patients with cardiomyopathia, end stage coronary disease or left ventricular assist device after heart surgery who are eligible for heart transplantation[9].

There are few differences between the European and the American guidelines in the definition and the management of heart failure. Acute heart failure due AHA/ACC guidelines is characterized by a rapid or gradual onset of signs and symptoms of heart failure, resulting in unplanned hospitalizations or office or emergency room visits [10].

The ESC guidelines state that acute heart failure is defined as the rapid onset of symptoms and signs, secondary to abnormal cardiac function [11,12]. The word "rapid" is part of both definitions but remains undefined and may mean hours, days or even a week or two [13]. The European guidelines advise the use of the measurement of brain natriuretic peptide as a screening test before proceeding to an echocardiogram whereas the US guideline simply recommends an echocardiogram in any patient.

The Guidelines of the American Heart Association (AHA) for the management of heart failure define four stages [10]. Patients with stage-A heart failure are at high risk of developing heart insufficiency due to conditions like hypertension, coronary artery disease, diabetes mellitus, a history of cardiotoxic drug therapy, alcohol abuse, a history of rheumatic fever or a family history of cardiomyopathy. These patients have no evidence of structural heart disease.
Patients with stage-B heart failure have structural heart disease such as myocardial infarction, left ventricular hypertrophy, fibrosis or LV dilatation or hypocontractility, or asymptomatic valvular heart disease but no signs of insufficiency. Stage-C diseased patients have recent symptoms of heart failure and structural heart disease. Patients with stage-D disease show symptoms of cardiac insufficiency at rest despite medical therapy. These patients may require specialized therapies like transplantation.

The definition according to the American Heart Association classifies heart failure into four stages, including patients who are at high risk for developing heart failure. This new classification is intended to complement the classical New York Heart Association (NYHA) functional classification of heart failure into Class I (asymptomatic), Class II (symptomatic on less than ordinary exertion), Class III (symptomatic on ordinary exertion), and Class IV (symptomatic at rest) [10].

Prevalence and incidence depend on age. The prevalence of heart failure in Germany is about 2 %[5]. This would mean that 16 millions of Germans are suffering from heart failure. Changes in age distribution and longer life of patients with heart diseases are expected to increase the prevalence of heart failure. The statistics of deaths of the year 2005 registered 48.184 deaths for cause of heart failure in Germany. This is about 1 % of the total costs of diseases in the same year[5]. Improved management of hypertension, diabetes, hypercholesterolemia and other risk factors for heart failure as well as advances in the treatment of acute coronary syndromes had influences on the epidemiology. This improved management has on the one hand allowed people to live longer with risk factors allowing them the time to develop heart insufficiency with an increased in the incidence. On the other hand, the management of risk factors has also prevented heart failure with the opposite effect on incidence and prevalence data. The aging of the population and greater physician awareness and availability of noninvasive imaging, leading to more frequent and accurate diagnoses may also have contributed to increasing incidence and prevalence. [14]

1.1.1 Prevention

Heart failure is multifactorial and many risk factors have direct and indirect influence on its development. Coronary artery disease, hypertension, dilated cardiomyopathy and valvular heart disease are the most common causes in both genders. A combination of Coronary artery disease and hypertension is present in many patients. [15]

Known risk factors for the development of cardiac insufficiency are including modifiable lifestyle characteristics as well as non-modifiable pathophysiologic characteristics such as age, sex, genetic factors, early life influences and a family history of premature cardiovascular disease. When a person develops cardiovascular disease these non-modifiable factors may continue to contribute to the progression of the disease.

C-reactive protein is strongly and independently associated with occurrence of heart failure in men. In women, the association is weaker and does not persist after accounting for established cardiovascular risk factors [16]. There is evidence that inflammation plays a role in the pathophysiology of heart failure. Lipoprotein-associated phospholipase A2 has pro-inflammatory properties and is associated with heart failure [17].

Important modifiable risk factors include smoking, hypertension, raised total cholesterol as well as other changes of the blood lipid levels, obesity, excess alcohol consumption, physical inactivity and diabetes. Some risk factors are known to be more important on the development of cardiovascular disease risk in women compared to men and vice versa [18]. Primary prevention programmes in many countries attempt to reduce the incidence of cardiovascular disease in campaigns trying to modify these risk factors.

The genetic factors may lead to a predisposition or increased susceptibility of individuals but are not yet fully identified. Adverse lifestyle factors seem to interact with genetic influences. Family history of cardiovascular disease is an important risk factor as well it is not clearly understood whether this is due to genetic or environmental factors. There is evidence for an increase in the risk of cardiovascular disease with age and some reports as well regarding differences in risk factors between sexes.

Structural and diastolic echocardiographic parameters are associated with all-cause mortality in an asymptomatic population. However, the evidence is still inadequate to support the usefulness of echocardiography for screening to identify asymptomatic individuals with preclinical ventricular dysfunction [19].

New data include the CARISMA study that investigated the use of implantable loop recorders for detecting life-threatening arrhythmias in patients with left ventricular insufficiency and found that brady- and ventricular tachy-arrhythmias predicted an adverse prognosis [20]. The TRENDS study showed that the burden of atrial fibrillation detected by pacemakers or defibrillators predicted the risk of embolic events but not with sufficient precision to justify changes in anti-thrombotic management [21]. The REVERSE study suggested that cardiac resynchronization therapy improves ventricular function and reduces morbidity even in patients with few or no symptoms of heart failure and may delay or prevent worsening heart failure [21].

A major risk factor seems to be a personal history of cardiovascular disease as this may indicate an individual susceptibility to the development of the disease as well as the possible presence of an underlying pathology like coronary artery stenosis. Overall it seems that risk factor intervention over the last decade has not been satisfying. Health promotion interventions result in only small changes in risk factors and mortality in the general population.

The SCORE (Systematic Coronary Risk Evaluation) project[22] has produced risk charts that are based on cholesterol, blood pressure and age for low-risk and high-risk European countries.
Major intervention trials with angiotensin-converting enzyme inhibitors or angiotensin receptor blockers have shown that these agents reduce the risk for cardiovascular events in patients at all levels of risk, with the greatest benefits seen in those at highest risk[4].

The predictive accuracy of the SCORE has been studied in a large Austrian population and though the SCORE-project overpredicted the mortality pattern in the cohort as a whole, its predictive ability at the individual level was classified as a useful utility in routine practice[23].
A comparison of the associations between risk factors and cardiovascular disease in Asia and Australasia showed that classical vascular risk factors act similarly in Asian and Caucasian populations and that prevention and treatment strategies should be similar[24].

The greatest benefits are generally obtained in secondary prevention i.e. after myocardial infarction or angina. Intervention in this group is likely to be more successful as the participants are more likely to change their behaviours. Thus it seems that risk factor intervention could be more successful if it is aimed at specific risk groups.

1.1.2 Prognosis

The prognosis of heart insufficiency in its natural course is bad, as shown by the outcomes of the classical Framingham-survey, and it is associated with a mortality of up to 50% in the first 5 years after the first cardiac decompensation [25,26]. More recently the Münster Heart Study (PROCAM) identified risk factors and assessed their relative importance by means of mathematical modelling[27].

The association between the NYHA classification and the outcome in heart failure has been studied and confirmed as a marker of hospitalization and mortality in ambulatory patients with chronic heart failure. Recently a mortality rate of 34% in NYHA classes I and II and 42% patients in NYHA classes III and IV has been published [28]. Hospitalizations due to all causes occurred in 66% in NYHA classes I and II and 71% in NYHA classes III and IV [28].

Heart failure accounts for 1 million hospital discharge diagnoses annually and a total mortality of over 260,000 in the USA. It is the leading cause of hospitalization, accounting for at least 20% of all hospitalizations in the patients over the age of 65 [29]. In longitudinal cohorts the 1-year survival in heart failure ranges from 55% to 90%, and 5-year survival ranges from 20% to 55%[26].

The Eurotransplant allocation algorithm, implemented in 2000, gives priority for heart transplantation to patients with high urgency status. This status is discontinued after a ventricular assist device implantation[30].

The prognosis of candidates for heart transplantation in the Eurotransplant heart allocation system has been analyzed for patients being listed with 'urgent status' for donor heart allocation or after ventricular assist device implantation without application for urgent status. The survival after listing for urgent status was significantly better than that in group with an assist device [31].

An implantable LV assist device has benefited patients with endstage heart failure as a bridge to cardiac transplantation. However, cardiac transplantation is not a viable option for the vast majority of patients with end-stage disease. 129 transplant-ineligible patients with a mean age of 67 years with end-stage cardiac insufficiency were randomized to medical therapy or to an LVAD [32]. The 2-year survival was 23% in the LVAD-treated group versus 8% in the medical-therapy–treated group. These data suggest using a LVAD as an alternative therapy in selected patients who are not candidates for cardiac transplantation.

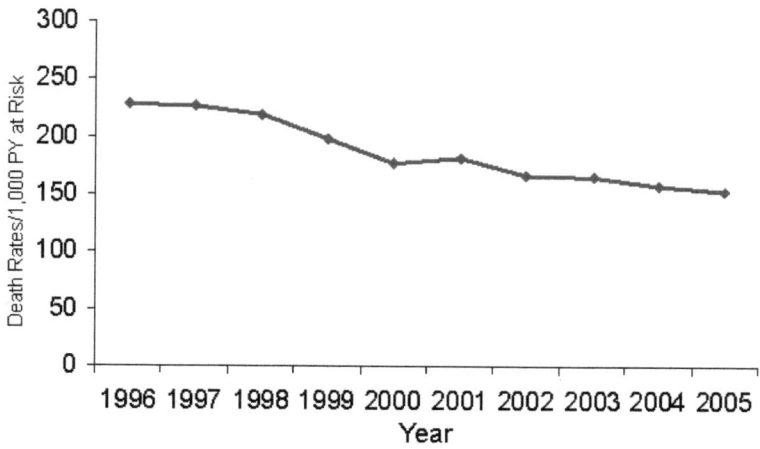

Fig 3: Annual death rate of patients on the waiting list for transplantation
Annual Report of the U.S. Organ Procurement and Transplantation Network
OPTH/SRTR 2006, Table 11.3

1.1.3 Therapy

Differences exist between European and American guidelines for the management of heart failure due to differences in health-care systems as well as there is little agreement on how to assess clinical trials and convey conclusions in a clear format [13].

Newer strategies of therapy like the introduction of the ACE-inhibitors still left a rather high mortality rate of 38% after a follow-up of 42 months. Overall, ACE inhibitor therapy significantly reduced the risk of the major clinical outcomes by 22% [33,34]. The Survival and Ventricular Enlargement (SAVE) study was designed to test the hypothesis that the use of angiotensin-converting enzyme inhibitors could prevent a further deterioration of ventricular function after myocardial infarction and improve the outcome. Regardless of the progress in conservative therapy of cardiac insufficiency, in the USA 35.000 patients per year have died from cardiac insufficiency in its final stage [35].

The treatment of stage-A disease is mainly the therapy of underlying conditions such as hypertension [10,36] and lipid disorders [10,37,38]; encourage regular exercise; discourage smoking and alcohol consumption. The use of ACE-inhibitors may be beneficial and educational programs may be needed [39,40]. The guidelines recommend for patients with stage-B disease the strategies described in stage-A and the treatment with ACE inhibitors and beta-blockers. General measure for treatment of stage-C heart failure consists of the identification of underlying causes. Myocardial ischemia should be treated with nitrates and beta-blockers. Any person without contraindications to coronary revascularization should have coronary angiography and percutaneous transluminal coronary angioplasty should be performed in selected patients. Anticoagulation might be needed. Regular physical activity should be encouraged in patients with mild-to-moderate heart disease. In end-stage heart failure an implantable left ventricular assist device (LVAD) might be indicated as a bridge to cardiac transplantation or as a permanent treatment option.

Currently, the orthotopic heart transplant is still the most effective treatment of terminal heart insufficiency with satisfying long-term results[41], although waiting periods to transplantation have to be overcome. In the case of cardiac decompensation occurring to patients on the waiting list, which cannot be controlled conservatively, patients have to be stabilised by mechanical pump systems until a suitable organ is available. As the number of transplantations is decreasing over the last years assist devices as destination therapy have become increasingly desirable. The limited availability of donor organs was also encountered by expanding the criteria for acceptable organs. Donor organs that wouldn't have been considered transplantable otherwise, particularly regarding donor-recipient size mismatching, are considered for transplant by carefully determining the risks of the patient [42,43].

Little information is available in the pediatric age group. Donor heart failure is referred to as the main cause of early mortality in pediatric heart transplantation. The use of oversized donor may be beneficial, particularly in patients with pretransplantation pulmonary hypertension. The use of undersized donor grafts should be strongly discouraged [43].

Donor-specific parameters that predict success or failure after heart transplantation are not defined. One analysis supports cautious extension of the criteria for donor acceptance but with an anticipated greater risk in the presence of a longer ischemic time, particularly in older donors given inotropic support [42]. The possibilities of expanding the pool of donor organs in generell are considered to be exhausted. A new development is the inclusion of "non-beating heart donors". Patients who are diagnosed 'brain stem dead' and have no pulse, therefore no heart beat, can donate tissues at various times after heart death. Typically these times vary from up to 24 hours for corneas to a maximum of 72 hours for heart valves. To enable the organs to be functioning they must have an oxygenated blood flow after death so the patient is on mechanical support at an ICU.

The COCPIT study [44] found a survival benefit from transplantation in German transplantation-candidates only for patients with a predicted high risk of dying on the waiting list. Patients with a predicted low or medium risk had no mortality risk reduction from transplantation; organ saving treatments have been recommended.

Many patients show contraindications for an organ transplant. With regard to the limited resources based on the chronic lack of donor organs, the development of alternatives to orthotopic heart transplants is necessary.

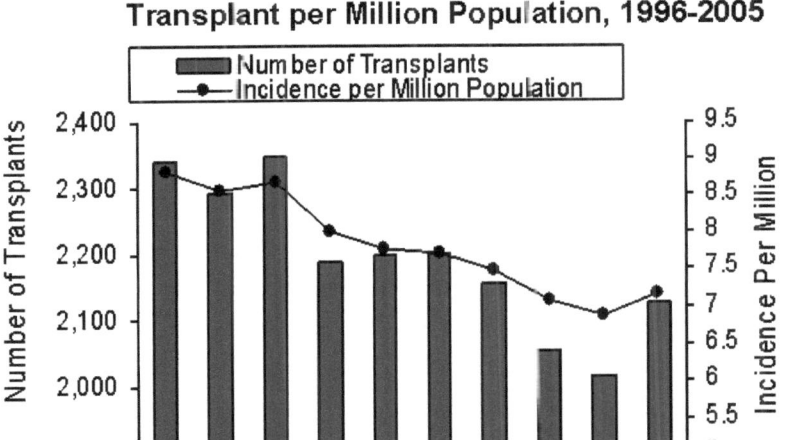

Fig 4: Heart transplants in the USA
Annual Report of the U.S. Organ Procurement and Transplantation Network
OPTH/SRTR 2006, Table 11.4

A number of different types of ventricular assist devices is available nowadays that can be implanted and partly or completely take over the cardiovascular function [45-48]. Device selection is based on little comparative data and mainly on the experience of the corresponding clinic; there are no recommendations available [45]. The use of ventricular assist devices has become a widely accepted therapeutic option. However, there are still limitations to the patient collective eligible for VAD placement such as acute renal failure, difficult psychosocial circumstances, signs of an infect during antibiotic therapy, coagulopathies in hepatic diseases, a patient after mechanical aortal valve replacement and ages over 70 years [47,48].

1.2 Types of support

A Ventricular assist device (VAD) is a mechanical pump system used to partially or completely replace the function of a failing heart. Ventricular assist devices may be used for a limited time frame, especially for patients as a bridge to transplantation or recovering from heart surgery and others are intended for long term or even life-long implantation in patients suffering from congestive heart failure[9,49].

VADs need to be clearly distinguished from artificial hearts, which are generally used after the removal of the patient's heart. It is distinct from a cardiopulmonary bypass, which is an external device that oxygenates the blood as well and therefore provides the function of both the heart and the lung. Artificial hearts have been used for long-term periods.

VADs differ from the total artificial heart as the biological heart is not removed[50]. Assist devices may include either a Left Ventricular Assist Device (LVAD) or a Right Ventricular Assist Device (RVAD) or both at once (BiVAD). Biventricular supporting systems may be extracorporeal situated devices which are pneumatically and pulsatile driven; they were the first assist devices that have been technically so well engineered that they achieved clinical application. The necessary size of the pneumatic driving unit implies a limited mobility of the treated patients[32,51,52].

The published indications for total artificial hearts include irreversible biventricular heart failure with a predicted life expectancy of less than 30 days, failure to respond to maximal medical therapy, age over 18 years, the patient is not eligible for heart transplantation and should have an acceptable surgical risk [50].

Indications for BiVAD Implantation include acute cardiogenic shock with multiorgan dysfunction with coagulopathy, intractable ventricular arrhythmia or persistent ventricular fibrillation, severe right ventricular dysfunction–characterized as a central venous pressure of greater than 18 mm Hg or a mean pulmonary arterial pressure above 25 mm Hg or diastolic pulmonary arterial pressure over 15 mm Hg on inotropic support; Giant cell myocarditis; acute biventricular myocardial infarction with or without ventricular septal defect; acute biventricular postcardiotomy failure and an LVAD flow <2.0 L/min/m2 and CVP >18mm Hg after LVAD implantation [51]. Biventricular systems are mostly applied in case of severe biventricular failures and in patients in cardiogenic shock with rapidly declining organ functions due to hypoperfusion or in advanced stages of organ failure[51,53].

In contrast to the total artificial heart the ventricular assist device provides only a part of the total cardiac output. The choice of which device should be used depends on the underlying disease and the pulmonary arterial resistance. In case of high pulmonary arterial resistance, a right ventricular assist may be necessary[52,54,55].

For univentricular support there are numerous different pumps available. Implantable LVADs have the great advantage of giving the patient a high degree of mobility and therefore provide a rather normal life in an ambulant treatment setting[56,57].
The European registry on clinical application of mechanical circulatory support systems reports the following indications for LVAD circulatory support as hemodynamic deterioration before transplantation, post acute myocardial infarction, postcardiotomy cardiogenic shock, graft failure and cardiac rejection [58].

Pumps used may be divided into two main categories - pulsatile pumps producing a physiologic pulse pattern and continuous flow pumps. In pulsatile systems blood is alternately sucked into the pump from the left ventricle then being forced out into the aorta. Continuous flow pumps use either centrifugal pumps or axial flow pump. Both types have a central rotor containing permanent magnets. In centrifugal pumps the rotors accelerate the blood moving it towards the outer rim whereas in axial flow pumps rotors are rather cylindrical with helical blades therefore accelerating the blood in the direction of the rotor's axis[59,60].

The implantation of artificial blood pumps for the treatment of terminal heart insufficiency has become at least at transplant clinics an established concept in treatment. As an assisted circulation often has to be maintained over months, the individual components of these life-supporting systems are subject to strong mechanical strain. As a fast change is usually not possible with blood pumps quite stable systems have been developed[61,62].

1.2.1 Pulsatile Systems

The pulsatile artificial ventricle rhythmically ejects a defined volume and therefore systolic as well as diastolic pressure can be measured in the circulation. Pulsatile systems have a synthetic blood sack which is incorporated in a casing; the systole is produced by compression, the input by suction or passive filling. The blood flow is directed by integrated valves. Due to their construction these systems are rather voluminous [63].

As patients have been supported for longer durations with paracorporal ventricular assist devices the need for implantable options increased. By implanting only the mechanically simple blood pump the control unit is remaining external where it can be serviced more easily. A small pneumatic driveline for the VAD is tunneled out of the body. The inner surfaces of the cannulas, as well as the blood sack in the ventricle are coated with heparin and should therefore reduce the thrombogenity of the artificial material [64]. Additional sizes of ventricles are available (up to 10ml for infants; normally 60-80 ml ventricles for adults) and therefore the application is possible for infants and children [65,66] although limited experience exists in this particular patient population.

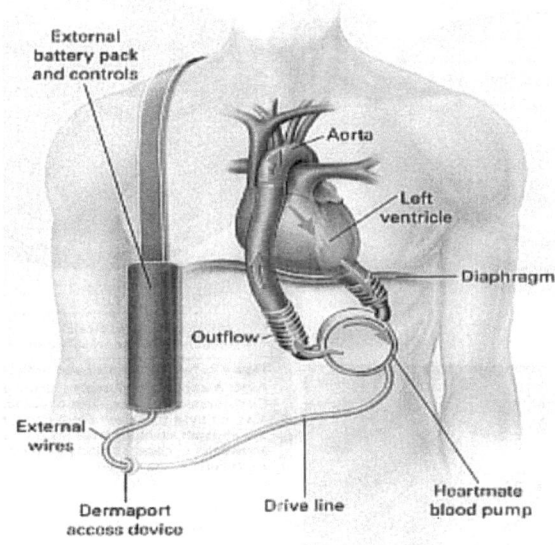

Fig 5: Example of a pulsatile pump in situ:
The HeartMate Assist Device implanted within the abdominal wall
Source: Columbia University College of Physicians & Surgeons;
Dept. of surgery

The device consists of an electric motor and a driveline. Blood fills the pump through a tube placed in the left ventricle and is being pumped into the aorta. When the diaphragm moves down, blood from the left ventricle again fills the pump.
These pumps may be implanted either paracorporally or intracorporally. In paracorporal systems the blood pump is situated outside of the body and connected to the heart and the large vessels via cannulas. These systems are implanted especially when short implantation periods are expected. They have the advantage of a lower incidence of sack infections however infections may develop alongside the cannulas. As the pumps lies paracorporally these systems can also be applied to small patients.

Intracorporal pumps are smaller and connected to a portable drive via a drive cable. The implantation of the ventricles takes place in a preperitoneal or intraperitoneal position [67]. Peritoneal placement may increase the risk that abdominal organs might be injured by direct contact with the pump.

The control system may remain extracorporally and can therefore easily be replaced in case of technical errors.

Types of pulsatile devices designed for children are the Thoratec device; the Novacor LVAD; the Medos-HIA system, which is driven pneumatically and is available in three different ventricular sizes of 10, 25, and 60 ml. For right ventricular support implantation of the 10% smaller sizes of 9, 22.5, and 54 ml have been reported [68].

There is increasing experience with the Berlin Heart VAD[64], which is available in different sizes of 10, 30, 50 and 80 ml with the smallest pump sizes suitable for infant support.

1.2.2 Continuous flow systems

Continuous flow is achieved by blood pumps designed similarly to turbines that cause a non-pulsatile blood flow pattern. The advantage of fully implantable axial pumps is their small size; therefore the implantation is less complex, the operation trauma is lower and so is the risk of bleeding and infections. Axial pumps consume little energy, they do not have an exhaust port or a pressure equalisation valve as compared to fully implanted pulsatile pumps; they are not as loud and incur fewer costs over time due to the reduction of possible device failures[59,60,69]. They are usually implanted over a median sternotomy, blood is drawn in over the apex of the left ventricle and re-infused into the aorta. Due to their small size they may also be implanted in small patients. Currently they are univentricularly deployed as LVADs but a biventricular full-implantation should be possible as well.

A single versatile part s in the pump ventricle, which rotates at a defined speed depending on the manufacturer. An ultrasound-flow-measure at the point of outflow continuously determines the blood flow. The electromagnetically driven motor is situated around the impeller [70,71].

After clinical trials of the MicroMed DeBakey VAD in November 1998 in Europe and in June 2000 in the United States the collected data supported the safety and performance of the device. Results show that the device is able to provide adequate circulatory support in patients with end-stage heart failure.

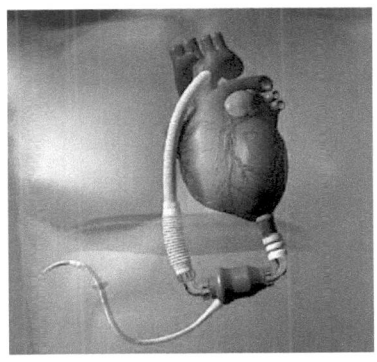

Fig 6. Example of a Rotary Blood Pump in situ
Source: Thoratec HeartMate®; Texas Heart Institute

1.3 Clinical used rotary pump systems

Different rotary pumps are available for the clinical application of mechanical assist devices and several new types of devices have been introduced in the last decades, i.e. the Vienna Artificial Heart in the Eighties, the Novacor portable system for home patients, the Micromed axial flow pump and the Arrow Lionheart.

In the year 2006 a total of 24 pumps have been implanted in the Department for Cardiothoracic Surgery at the Medical University of Vienna, the used systems were the Thoratec VAD (2), the MicroMed DeBakey-VAD (15), the HeartWareHVAD (4), the Novacor LVAS (2) and the Berlin Heart Incor (1). [72]

The major advantage of rotary pumps is their smaller size compared to pulsatile systems, their biocompatibility and the soundlessness during operation. Axial-flow left ventricular assist devices are simpler, smaller, and easier to operate than are pulsatile pumps.

BLOOD PUMPS

Pulsatile VAD	Rotary Blood Pumps			Total Artificial Heart
	Axial Pumps	Radial Pumps	Diagonal Pumps	
HeartMate	Hemopump	Biopump	Caplox SP	Ventr. Assist	Heart Quest	Abiomed TAH	Akutsu III
LionHeart	Sun Waseda	Delphin	Isoflow	DeltaStream	HIA	Cardiowest	Liotta TAH
Medos	HeartMate II	CorAide	GyroPump			PennState TAH	Utah TAH
BVS 500	Valvo Pump	RotaFlow	HIFlow			Philadelphia Heart	Nimbus TAH
Toyobo	Jarvik 2000	Nikkiso Pump	AB-180			Baylor TAH	Undulation Pump
BCM	DeBakey	Vienna Cent.	Evaheart				
Roller Pump	Impella	Abiomed CF	Kriton Pump				
HeartSaver	Streamliner	MSCP	Heart Mate III				
Novacor							
Thoratec							
Berlin Herat							
Nippon Zeon							
Alvad							
Cora Pump							
IA Balloonp.							
PUCA							

Fig 7: Overview on different blood pump systems [73]

Third-generation blood pumps are using the magnetic-levitation system, which can be categorized into three types: external motor-driven system, direct-drive motor-driven system and self-bearing motor system[74].

1.3.1 The DuraHeart System

The Dura Heart consists of an implantable Pump and several components that support the function of the Pump. In this external motor-driven system the impeller is levitated in the axial or z-direction. The disadvantage of this system is the mechanical wear in the mechanical bearings of the external motor. The system consists of a titanium pumping unit, a titanium inflow and outflow conduit, and a drive and control console. A displacement volume of 180 mL, a weight of 540 g, an external diameter of 72 mm, and a height of 45 mm were attained, allowing the pump to be implanted in the patients with a body surface area of less than 1.1 m^2. The pumping unit consists of an upper housing with the levitation system, impeller, and bottom housing. Three electromagnets and three position sensors are mounted in the upper housing. Tilting and axial displacements of the impeller are monitored and controlled using a three-DOF control. A levitated impeller is driven through a magnetic coupling force from the direct current brushless motor mounted outside. Radial impeller movement is passively suspended with a bias flux through electromagnetic rotor and drive magnet rotor. The pump speed is controlled from 1200 to 2600 rpm and can produce a flow rate of 2–10 L/min. The clinical implant of the DuraHeart left ventricular assist system was started in January 2004 in Bad Oeynhausen. [74]

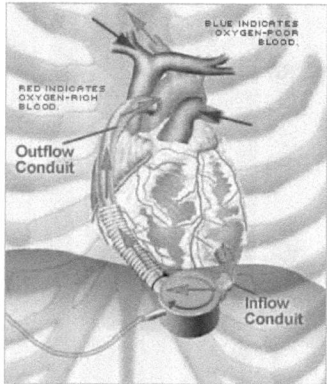

Fig. 8: DuraHeart® left ventricular assist device[74].

1.2.3 The Berlin Heart

In this system the impeller is made into the rotor of the motor and the magnetic flux rotates the impeller. Axial impeller movement is monitored by a position sensor and controlled actively by the two electromagnets mounted at both ends of the rotor. Radial and tilting impeller movements are passively controlled. Levitated impeller can be rotated at speeds between 5000 and 10 000 rpm generating up to 5 L/min of flow against a pressure of 100 mm Hg. The motor efficiency of more than 90% and power consumption <4 W ensure that the pump does not generate any significant amount of heat. The control software enables monitoring of the pressure gradient and the flow by detection of the rotor's position in the magnetic field. An antisuction algorithm can be activated to eliminate suction of ventricular structures. The pump, which is made of titanium, weighs 200 g, has an axial direction of 120 mm, an outer diameter of 30 mm, and a volume of 80 mL. The pump is controlled through a percutaneous cable connected to the control unit and a main as well as a backup battery. The flow straighter and diffuser are adapted for inflow and outflow passage, respectively, to reduce the spin of blood flow and add to the pressure buildup. The first human clinical trial was started 2002, at the German Heart Institute, Berlin, Germany. [74]

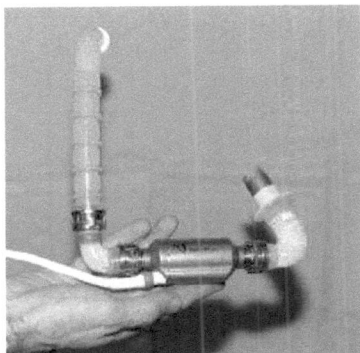

Fig. 9: The Berlin Heart Incor®

1.2.3 The HeartMate II

The Heart Mate II LVAD is a small and quiet rotary pump with a single-moving part which makes it possible to provide long-term circulatory support [75]. The clinical outcome includes low thrombosis, low hemolysis, and low infection rates[76]. Of the 43 patients in this study where the HeartMate II was implanted 35 were discharged from the hospital.

The HeartMate II has a left ventricular apical inflow cannula with a sintered titanium blood-contacting surface. The bladed impeller spins on a bearing and is powered by an electromagnetic motor. No compliance chamber or valves are necessary, and a single driveline exits the right lower quadrant of the abdomen. The inlet cannula is placed in the ventricular apex and the pump is placed either intraperitoneally or extraperitoneally. The outflow cannula is connected to a Dacron graft, which is then anastomosed to the ascending aorta. The external controller and batteries resemble those of the original HeartMate as well. The pump is designed to spin at 6,000 to 15,000 rpm and to deliver as much as 10 L/min of cardiac output. A computerized algorithm is used to continuously estimate flow from the device. [77]

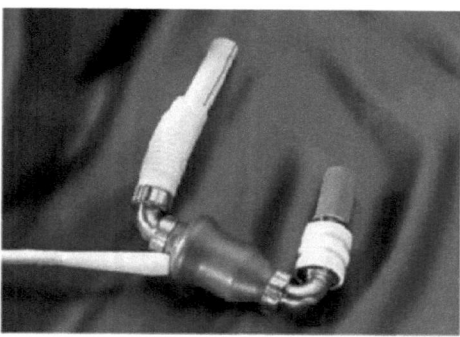

Fig.10: HeartMate® II left ventricular assist device[78].

1.3.4 The MicroMed DeBakey VAD

The electromagnetically actuated DeBakey VAD is a miniaturized, fully implantable titanium axial-flow blood pump. A titanium inflow cannula connects the pump to the apex of the left ventricle and a vascular graft as an outflow conduit connects the pump to the ascending aorta. An ultrasonic flow probe is placed around the outflow conduit. Together with the flow probe's wiring, the pump motor cable exits the skin and attaches to the VAD's external controller system.

The pump is designed to achieve 5 L/min against 100 mm Hg pressure, with a rotor speed of 7500-12500 rpm and a power input of 10 W. The measured pump flow is displayed either on the external VAD controller or when connected on the clinical data acquisition system together with pump speed, power consumption, and current signals from the pump.

Adjustments to the pump speed can be performed only when it is connected to the data acquisition system. The power can be delivered by two 12-V batteries for several hours. [79]. The length is 76,2 mm and the diameter 30,5 mm.

The development of the DeBakey VAD Child from MicroMed Technology, Inc is reducing the technological gap between adults and children. [80] The first clinical trials were started in 1998 in Berlin and Vienna. The DeBakey VAD® Child by MicroMed Technology, Inc., Houston, TX, USA became available in February 2004[80]. This pediatric device employs the same axial flow pump that is used in the adult version[81].

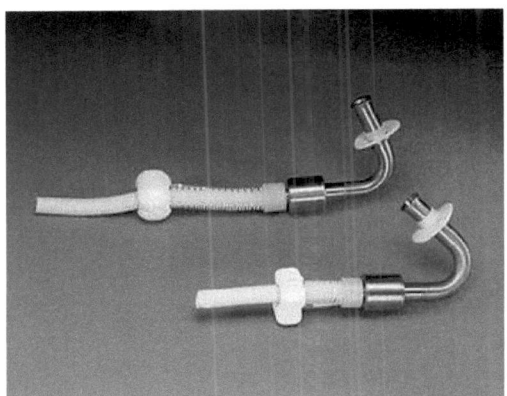

Fig. 11: MicroMed DeBakey VAD® left ventricular assist device.

1.3.5 The HeartWare Left Ventricular Assist Device

The HeartWare Left Ventricular Assist Device is a small centrifugal blood pump capable of generating up to 10 litres per minute of forward flow. The pump is designed to draw blood from the apex of the left ventricle and to propel it through an outflow graft connected to the patient's ascending aorta. With a displaced volume of 45cc this pump is designed to be implanted in the pericardial space directly adjacent to the heart and above the diaphragm. Implantation above the diaphragm is expected to lead to short surgery time and quick recovery.

The pump has only one moving part, the impeller, which spins at rates between 2,000 and 3,000 revolutions per minute. The impeller is suspended within the pump housing through a combination of passive magnets and a hydrodynamic thrust bearing. This hydrodynamic suspension is achieved by a gentle incline on the upper surfaces of the impeller blades. When the impeller spins, blood flows across these inclined surfaces, creating a "cushion" between the impeller and the pump housing. There are no mechanical bearings or any points of contact between the impeller and the pump housing. The pump's inflow cannula is integrated with the device itself, ensuring proximity between the heart and the pumping mechanism. The use of a wide-bladed impeller and the clear flow paths through the system are expected to help minimize any risk of pump induced hemolysis or thrombus. The first clinical implantation was 2006 in Vienna.

The HeartWare System is currently the subject of an international clinical trial involving five investigational centres in Europe and Australia. Patient enrolment in the trial was completed in August 2007. [78]

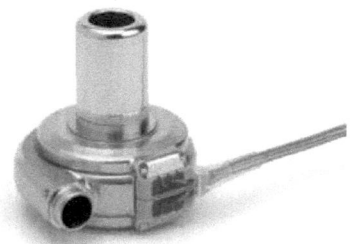

Fig.12: HeartWare left ventricular assist device[78].

1.3.6 VentrAssist LVAD

The VentrAssist is a new third generation cardiac assist system primarily designed as a permanent alternative to heart transplants. VentrAssist has a hydrodynamically suspended impeller as moving part. It weighs 298 grams and measures 60mm in diameter, making it suitable for both children and adults.

The implanted parts of the VentrAssist device use materials which are fully biocompatible including titanium alloys. The benefits are the biocompatibility and the absence of wearing parts as well as an advanced information management to log critical data[82]. The VentrAssist incorporates a third-generation centrifugal pump featuring the hydrodynamic suspension of an "open-flow" rotor. This design allows blood to flow through the center of the rotor and over its outer surface, thus maximizing washing of all blood-contacting surfaces. Thrombosis risk has been minimized by the use of a diamond-like carbon coating on the blood contacting surfaces of the pump and a blood flow path designed to ensure all areas within the pump are washed, with no areas of stasis, flow obstruction, or retrograde flow. Connection to the left ventricular apex is by a short silicone inflow cannula with a bell-shaped end. The outflow is connected to the ascending aorta by a polyester graft. Two externally-worn batteries and a compact controller provide power to the implanted pump by a 6.4-mmdiameter percutaneous lead. The clinical studies in Europe are finished and ongoing in the United States.

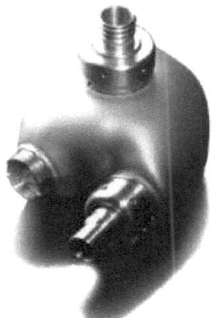

Fig.13: VentrAssist LVAD[82]

1.4 Indications

1.4.1 Rescue support

Rescue support stands for a mechanical support of the cardiovascular system for hours or days in order to enable fast myocardial recovery.

The main indication for rescue treatment is cardiac insufficiency after cardiotomy which makes it impossible to avoid a cardiopulmonary bypass. The incidence after cardio-surgical procedures is about 0.5-1% of the patients [83]. Usually highly dosed catecholamines and an intraaortic balloon pump are applied. If it's still not possible to establish a sufficient cardiac output one has to consider an assist-implantation taking the contra-indications into account. If it is possible to achieve an acceptable cardiac output at first but myocardial recovery in the post-surgical course is not observable and the patient remains in the low-cardiac-output-syndrome, the indication for an assist-implantation may be given again [83]. Successful support has allowed for myocardial recovery and survival in several settings of intractable cardiogenic shock.

1.4.2 Bridge to heart transplant

Bridge to heart transplant can be defined as mid- to longterm cardiovascular support for days or months of transplant candidates until a suitable donor organ can be implanted. In this context an emergency and an elective assist-implantation can be distinguished.

Bridge to transplant (BTT) is indicated if no suitable transplant is available for the patient in cardiogenic shock. The implantation of an artificial pump can lead to stabilisation and mobilisation of the patient. The patient is kept alive by an assist device until an acceptable donor organ is found. The period of this time is variable; durations of up to one year are not unusual[56].

Congestive heart failure is a progressive disease despite newer therapy options some patients remain severely symptomatic. It should be regarded if therapy really fails or whether the treatment is not increased sufficiently. An increase in serum creatinine up to 30-50%, hyperkaliemia up to 5.5 mmol/l, and asymptomatic hypotension and bradycardia are usually acceptable [84]. If patients remain severely symptomatic despite adequate medical therapy heart transplantation is indicated if no other therapeutic options are effective and there are no contraindications. In these patients assist devices might be used as bridge to transplant if the medical therapy leads to a minimum of cardiac function.

The current indications for long-term mechanical support as bridge to transplantation first require the patient to be a transplant candidate. Patients need to be listed for a heart transplant before the implantation of some of these devices. This may be a very difficult decision as mechanical support can be used to support a patient to make him a transplant candidate what he otherwise would not have been. If the patient were subsequently determined to not be a good surgical candidate he may be, supported with the LVAD as destination therapy [49].

Bridging to transplant with a left ventricular assist device can be limited by severe right ventricular failure, although survival can be improved with early right-ventricular device insertion [85].

The emergency indication is provided for patients with acute or chronic terminal heart insufficiency when hemodynamics worsens rapidly despite maximum inotropic therapy. The clinical challenge is to choose patients with imminent ischemic organ damage for an assist-implantation in time so irreversible organ damages can be prevented.

The more elective indication allows for the implantation of transplant candidates, who, under maximum conservative therapy, have sufficient cardiovascular circumstances. Whether transplant results themselves can additionally be improved by assist-device implantation due to patient recovery remains to be clarified [56,86,87]. Risk factor analysis in this group revealed that previous heart surgery, infective pneumonia, shock-related coagulation disorders and an age greater than 50 years may have an unfavourable influence on patient survival. Reliable prediction of outcome in the bridge to transplantation group requires further experience.

1.4.3 Bridge to myocardial recovery

Temporary heart failures with a perspective for recovery are indications for bridge to recovery. In some patients myocardial function can recover within weeks or months to the extent that the assist device can be explanted successfully. Myocardial recovery has been described in patients with acute myocarditis and dilative or ischemic cardiomyopathy [88-90]. It has been shown that even a striking degree of myocardial fibrosis can reduce to normal values after explantation of the device and may be an indicator for outcome. The echcardiographic parameter left ventricular diameter in diastole and left ventricular ejection fraction served as the main parameters to assess changes in cardiac performance.

After recovery of the myocardial function, the patient can be weaned from the cardiovascular support and the assist device can be explanted.
A stable long-term course after bridge to recovery therapies has been documented sufficiently [91,92]. The mechanical unloading during left ventricular assist device support may lead to cardiac recovery. Predictors of recovery, however, have not been identified but echocardiographic, ECG, histologic, and neurohormonal improvement during LVAD support has been published [93]. Cardiac recovery peaked by 60 days, and there was a trend toward progressive improvement in QRS duration with ongoing support. Complete cardiac recovery may be achieved in case of early posttransplant graft failure.

The achievability of device weaning in patients receiving left ventricular assist devices as a bridge to transplantation has been studied [57]. During a four-month follow-up, patients were evaluated with right heart catheterization and echocardiography and studied with the device turned off. Patients with severe advanced heart failure were unlikely to show significant cardiac recovery following treatment in this study.

Anyway patients with end-stage heart failure placed on a cardiac assist device may show at least some degree of improvement of cardiac function.

It has been shown that left ventricular assist devices with continuous flow have similar pre- and posttransplant outcomes in terms of pre- and posttransplant mortality in comparison with pulsatile LVADs [94]. However, the rate and severity of posttransplant rejection was higher in the group with continuous flow devices [94].

In a subgroup of selected patients, weaning from the device offers an alternative to cardiac transplantation; in these patients the transplantation could be no longer necessary. This may save donor hearts and is preferred to cardiac transplant. However no reliable single parameter predicts outcome after weaning or determines the possibility of device removal before implantation in advance[91].

Further studies of the timing of the LVAD implantation and explantation, adjunct medical therapy and optimum weaning strategies might help to improve the success. Heart insufficiency is likely to reoccur in 25% of the cases after weaning from the assist device and the development over time is hardly predictable. The probability that the patient can be weaned from the VAD is better in younger patients and in fast recovery of the myocardial function with the assist device[95].

1.4.4 Permanent assist device

Alternative to transplant (ATT) is a term used in case that the irreversible damaged heart can be functionally replaced by an artificial device. The assist device remains implanted permanently as a destination therapy. Infection arising from the drive lines is a limiting factor in long-term use of the device in these patients. The use of the current available device for a longer time period should be reserved for patients for whom no other form of life support is available and for patients with contraindications for heart transplantation.

The classical Randomized Evaluation of Mechanical Assistance for the Treatment of Congestive Heart Failure (REMATCH) trial first demonstrated that implantation of left ventricular assist devices as destination therapy may provide survival superior to any known medical treatment in patients with end-stage heart failure who are ineligible for transplantation. The appropriate selection of candidates and timing of the implantation of the device are critical for improving the outcomes. Patients with advanced heart failure who are referred for destination therapy before major complications of heart failure develop have the best chance of achieving an excellent 1-year survival with LVAD therapy [62,96].

Left ventricular assist device failure rates are critical for their establishment as a long-term therapy for end-stage heart failure patients. Despite the observed rates of device malfunction and replacement, LVAD implantation contributes clinically significant improvement with regard to survival as compared with medical management [54,97]. Device modifications and innovations for infection management may improve the performance.

For these patients with an LVAD in situ, there was a trend for quality of life and psychological functioning to be poorer than for transplanted and explanted patients [61]. Psychological assessment and interventions to reduce psychological morbidity will be important in these patients, particularly in view of the possibility of their use for long-term destination therapy.

If the artificial organ should take over the entire heart function and the insufficient heart has been removed before the implantation it is called total artificial heart. Meanwhile assist devices are designed for long-term

application and further experience will show if they will develop to an accepted alternative to heart transplants.
Although the outcomes of device therapy are still limited by device durability and complications, the potential of the destination therapy should continue to expand through the development of newer, smaller, and more innovative ventricular assist devices [96,98].

1.5 Contraindications

Generally accepted contraindications for assist device implantation are irreversible damages of the central nervous system, an advanced hepatic disease, an irreversible pulmonary failure, uncontrollable blood coagulation, sepsis and a malign disease. Relative contraindications are acute renal failure, difficult psychosocial circumstances, signs of an infect during antibiotic therapy, coagulopathies in hepatic diseases, a patient after mechanical aortal valve replacement and ages over 70 years [56,83].

Although extensive studies have been done the selection of those patients being the best candidates for LVAD placement is still difficult. However, a number of absolute contraindications to LVAD implantation are known. These include issues like a small body surface area as well as active infection, an untreated malignant disease or another systemic illness likely to limit survival, severe and irreversible major organ dysfunction including significant aortic valve regurgitation [99]. In the REMATCH trial, some of these contraindications, such as previous malignancy have not been considered an absolute contraindication but have been weighed in relation to the expected survival of the patient. With growing clinical experience in dealing with assist devices the generally accepted contraindications are being discussed as well.

For patients who are designated for rescue support due to a cardiac failure after cardiotomy it is critical to define whether the cardio surgical procedure was successful and if there is a realistic chance for recovery of the myocardial function. The need for postcardiotomy mechanical support is reported to have a low incidence of 0.5%. The overall survival rate was 35%, but significantly better (72%) in the subgroup with an implantable system and later being bridged to transplantation [100].

For patients with bridge to heart transplants, the possibility of a transplant has to be evaluated and their agreement to the heart transplant should be obtained before the elective assist-device implantation. The pulmonary vascular resistance and the trans-pulmonary gradient have to be in an acceptable range for transplant and, if necessary, the reversibility of a pulmonary hypertension may be tested pharmacologically[101], but even a fixed pulmonary hypertension has shown to be possibly reversible [102,103]. In case of emergency indication a fast decision is usually made based on the clinical data.

1.6 Complications

Numerous problems have accompanied the development of assist device systems and are still being discussed.

Left ventricular assist device-associated complications can be broadly divided by their temporal occurrence. Early complications include perioperative hemorrhage, air embolism, infection, multi-organ failure and right ventricular failure. Most of the complications in LVAD patients are occurring in the perioperative time period and are the major causes of early mortality. These complication rates lower with experience and design improvement.

Long-term mortality is mostly related to the device dysfunction, infectious complications and thromboembolism. Improved understanding of the mechanisms involved should aid the clinician in further reducing the incidence of these occurrences[104].

The International Society for Heart and Lung Transplantation (ISHLT) has set a proposal for clinical standards for destination therapy programs, including a minimum set of requirements for training of physicians, surgeons, and other key personnel, and measurement of center-specific outcomes on an annual basis with continued approval based on achieving target outcomes.

The possibility of thromboembolic complications requires exact coagulation management usually with Coumarine sometimes in combination with aggregation inhibitors [105]. This may cause bleedings even after minimal traumas but very rarely severe cerebral bleedings. Left-ventricular assist device implantation is still associated with thromboembolism as the optimal anticoagulation is still unclear. Addition of platelet inhibitors to may help to prevent thromboembolism. Platelet inhibitors should be postponed until sufficient hemostasis is achieved as too early administration is associated with an increased risk of bleeding [106].

Renal failure and the multi-organ dysfunction syndrome (MODS) remain important causes of death; many patients are at time of implantation in a reduced state. Multiple organ dysfunction syndrome is the presence of altered organ function in acutely ill patients that may involve two or more organ systems. In some patients the artificial normalisation of the perfusion does not lead to a stabilisation of decompensated organ function. Infections, especially in the post surgical phase, can develop to a life threatening state. Infection of the VAD, which is often caused by Staphylococcus aureus, poses a major threat to survival [107].

Axial blood pumps have certain specific problems in common. Suction or emptying of the left ventricle can lead to an inflow obstruction or to a collapse of the ventricle – especially with hypovolemia or right ventricular failure [108,109].

Patients may develop secondary pulmonary hypertension due to their primary disease. This increase in the pulmonary vascular resistance can cause a failure of the right heart with consecutive low-cardiac-output syndrome and may be lowered after the implantation of an LVAD [102]. Nevertheless it could be demonstrated that the implantation of an LVAD supports the circulation of patients with terminal cardiac insufficiency effectively and that univentricular support can be applied successfully to a majority of the patients with biventricular cardiac insufficiency [110-112]. The need for excessive inotropic support while on the left ventricular support system appeared to be related to the elevated pulmonary vascular resistance in combination with large preimplantation ventricular volumes. It appears that even patients with compromised right ventricular performance can be supported long term with a left ventricular assist device.

Even if the pulmonary-arterial pressures and the pulmonary vascular resistance are carefully considered right ventricular dysfunction is common after LVAD implantations and cannot be precisely predicted.

Right ventricular dysfunction significantly affects mortality and morbidity after left ventricular assist device implantation. A dilated right ventricle with increased preload and afterload predisposes to a dysfunction. A main determinant, which decides over the survival after an LVAD implantation is the ability of the right ventricle to produce enough output in order to fill the LVAD [55]. Patients with elevated pulmonary vascular resistance may require temporary right ventricular support. One analysis revealed that right ventricular function significantly predicted left ventricular assist pump fill volume during the first 48 hours of support [113].

1.7 Trends and developments

Surgical treatment of patients with congestive heart failure has advanced from the first clinical application of left ventricular assist devices for patients with end-stage heart failure and the indications for their use have been increased. In the future further changes in the technology and patient selection are to be expected. Successful LVADs will have to show an excellent durability, be user-friendly and costeffective.

The objective of the initial phase of mechanical and pharmacologic therapy is to reverse ventricular remodelling possibly leading to a reversal of the reduced myocardial function. Device modifications and innovations for infection management exhibit new possibilities of improving device performance in the near future.

Strategies suggest adjunctive therapies in conjunction with the ventricular decompression by the LVAD adding 2-adrenergic receptor to stimulate left ventricular hypertrophy [114]. The application of cell transplantation and gene therapy to alter apoptosis seems to have benefits in mechanical ventricular decompression [115].

The increasing reliability may allow implantation at an easier stage of cardiac deterioration as doubts about the feasibility of long-term pulseless circulation are more and more disappearing. The newest developments including miniaturization, low power use, and ease of implantation are beginning to be shown in practice. This use as destination therapy in healthier patients would probably improve long-term morbidity and mortality, therefore the inclusion of patients in NYHA class III might be considered [114].

The indication for use in newborns and infants are likely to increase. Those heart surgeons who don't have these systems at their disposal will have to use ECMOs alternatively for infants as a mechanical support [95].

In the long run it is imaginable that the implantation of an assist device might replace medicinal therapy of terminal heart insufficiency which implies sufficient clinical experience and failure-free functioning assist devices over years [112]. The implantable left ventricular assist device was designed to provide circulatory support as an alternative to heart transplantation, so that questions regarding long-term device reliability and the chronic risk of infection are unknown.

2. Physiology of Reduced Pulsatility

The phenomenon of pulse-less or low-pulse circulation with the use of rotary blood pumps raises several questions concerning physiology. In fact a low pulsatility is observed in patients with rotary blood pumps, mainly after cardiac recovery [116,117]. Rotary pumps unload the left ventricle and decrease the end-diastolic diameter which may contribute to heart recovery. This unloaded left ventricle may provide a pulsatile flow in addition to the continuous flow of the assist device, this pulsatility is independent of peripheral vascular resistance. The VAD unloads the left ventricle which leads to a decrease in the end-diastolic left ventricular diameter and to the restoration of ventricular function. The unloaded left ventricle and the partially recovered right ventricle are after recovery able to provide an almost physiological pulsatile flow despite the continuous flow of the support. Unloading of the left ventricle leads to a change in the geometry of the right ventricle and an improvement in right ventricular function. Attempts to quantify pulsatility have been made [118,119]. A true flatline flow can be achieved only by running the pump on maximal support which might be dangerous due to a collapse of the left ventricle and should be prevented.

These pumps themselves generate a continuous blood flow which is different from the physiological condition of the beating heart. Although the flow pattern is usually not pulseless due to the remaining contractility of the supported left ventricle it is less pulsatile compared to the healthy heart. A pulse pressure is transmitted to the systemic circulation from the unloaded left ventricle.

The unloaded left ventricle provides pressure changes at the pump inlet as well therefore accelerating the flow through the pump and inducing pulsatile flow in the outflow. Pulsatility may occur even when the aortic valve remains closed and is not dependent on pump flow, blood pressure or systemic vascular resistance [59]. Axial pumps are sensitive to the differential pressure across the pump and therefore the afterload.

Typical values of flow observed in the early postoperative phase are in the range of 3–5 L/min resulting in a pressure difference of typically 5–15 mmHg. This flow and pressure pulsatility usually increases after recovery of the decompensated heart, but never regains the physiological pulsatility levels [116,120]. The performance of rotary pumps is proportional to rotor speed and inversely proportional to pressure differences across the inlet and outlet orifices of the pump. Rotary pumps have a potential capacity to adjust flow to changes in preload.

Numerical simulation studies of the carotid artery have been carried out and it was found that a washout phenomenon leads to only 20% extension of particle residence time under full pump support [121].

The classical REMATCH trial demonstrated a rather disappointing survival advantage for the HeartMate left ventricular assist device over medical treatment and stressed the risk of mechanical with the use of the first-generation technology[32]. Overall it seems that in patients receiving mechanical cardiac support survival seems to depend more on the condition of the patients and the reversibility of myocardial pathology than on the type of assist device employed [59].

2.1 Effects on the circulation

It has been assumed that assistence of the ventricle is most effective when there is enough remaining myocardial function to maintain at least some pulsatility to allow a reinstitution of the Frank-Starling response. In studies done in animals perfused by non-pulsatile flow [122] it has been assumed that a certain period of time was required to accommodate to this type of circulation. On the other hand it has been shown that the physiologic reaction to an immediate switch from pulsatile to nonpulsatile flow that most of the parameters did not differ from control levels after the switch indicating a good accommodation to nonpulsatile flow[123].

Elevation of plasma catecholamine levels immediately after the start of nonpulsatile flow decreased to normal 2 weeks later; serum catecholamine level did not change in stable hemodynamics [124,125]. As the continuous flow begins there is an acute vascular response with the release of renin [59]. This adrenergic response to absence of pulse pressure is more marked at low flows. Only a few long-term studies on the effects of nonpulsatile blood flow are available; but the existing evidence suggests that pulse pressure might not be required from a blood pump. End-organ function is well maintained with nonpulsatile systems.

A marked physiologic difference between pulsatile and non-pulsatile cardiac support could not be found even with an increased flow [122]. No long term influence on hemodynamics, oxygen consumption or blood catecholamines was demonstrated [123]. The required pump flow was within the same range as the flow required for pulsatile systems [116,117]. Mean blood pressure was not significantly different[69].

Major arteries are exposed to more than 100.000 pulse waves per day. The arterial structure is modified by changes in arterial pressure and blood flow [126]. The cyclic stretching during the pulse waves causes a proliferation. Nishimura evaluated aortic wall changes using a chronic nonpulsatile left heart bypass modeland showed that the wall thickness of aortic specimens are thinner[127]. The distribution of elastin and collagen has been estimated by a computed imaging system. This thinning of the medial layer of the aorta has been demonstrated but no functional changes could be found, the changes in the aortic wall do not cause significant changes in mechanical stiffness. The wall thickness of the aorta was found to be thinner with nonpulsatile left-heart support [127]. The results of this group indicated that prolonged nonpulsatile left heart bypass did not affect the vascular tonus but significantly diminished the vascular contractility. Media degeneration was found by other studies as well [69].

The arteries usually regulate perfusion by rapid contraction and relaxation of smooth muscle. Nishimura has investigated the pulse wave velocity during both pulsatile and nonpulsatile left heart bypass and showed no significant difference between the two systems [127]. The reason for the stability in mechanical properties may be the adaptation of arterial structure to the reduced pulse pressure. This group also reported that the systemic vascular resistance response to norepinephrine infusion decreased in prolonged nonpulsatile circulation. Prolonged continuous-flow left-heart bypass caused a decrease in systemic vascular resistance response to phenylephrine thus indicating a decrease of vasoconstrictive function.

One study demonstrated that pulsatile flow is associated with a better peripheral vascular reactivity than continuous flow an patients
supported by axial flow devices should be kept on the lowest speed setting to allow a maximum of pulsatility [128]. Shear stress may be important for thrombus formation. The nfluence of rotary blood pump support on shear stress patterns and streamlines has been demonstrated in a 3-dimensional model of the carotid artery[123]. To describe the blood flow a mathematical model for Newtonian fluids has been used in this study and the local effect

of continuous flow has been described as rather minimal with an existing stenosis. This has been shown previously for intact arterial geometries[121]. Usually coronary and myocardial blood flow is decreased during ventricular fibrillation compared with the beating heart [129]. A study on the effects on coronary perfusion and regional myocardial blood flow showed an increase in the resistance of the small vessels as well as a decrease of myocardial oxygen consumption and no histological changes have been observed [130].

Chronic nonpulsatile circulation does not alter peripheral perfusion or oxygen metabolism[131]. Recent studies have shown no difference in myocardial high-energy phosphate metabolism between pulsatile and nonpulsatile flow [59]. The peripheral circulatory changes have been studied with the use of thermography and a laser tissue flow meter in the auricle. Nonpulsatile flow maintained tissue perfusion in the normal range, the capillary flow had an intermittent vasomotion with a frequency of 10-20 ml/min. This suggests a capillary autoregulation maintaining appropriate regional blood flow[131,132]. It has been shown that continuous flow may produce an increase in cardiac vagal activity [133].

The interaction between left ventricle and continuous cardiac assist, the effect of different working conditions and support levels on left ventricular pressure-volume loop was investigated in acute animal experiments. PV loop analysis in continuous cardiac assist reveals that the endsystolic volume index and the enddiastolic volume index are strongly correlated and that endsystolic volume index varies considerably with preload [134].

Excessive ventricular unloading of the left ventricle during continuous left ventricular support can induce ventricular arrhythmias. Evidence supporting an increase in arrhythmic activity after suction has been detected, but it has turned out to be a transient effect, which vanished within 5 minutes after suction. ECG events related to suction have a sudden onset and are severe ventricular arrhythmias, which can consist of even just one extrasystolic beat, and they usually cease after clearance of suction [135].

Cardiac function recovers to some degree for most patients after VAD implantation. The molecular, cellular, biochemical, and structural changes occurring in the myocardium, often referred to as remodeling, have been studied extensively in patients with heart failure[136]. A specific pattern of expression of sarcomeric and non-sarcomeric proteins in the myocardium is thought to be essential for normal myocardial function.

A major feature of remodeling is that at some of its manifestations can be reversed. There is some evidence that prolonged unloading of the left ventricle with the use of a left ventricular assist device is associated with structural reverse remodeling that can be accompanied by functional improvement. Sufficient recovery to permit explantation of the device has been observed in 5 to 24% of patients[137]. Some drugs are known to enhance reverse remodeling, like the β2-adrenergic–receptor agonist clenbuterol[137].

A combination therapy consisting of unloading of the ventricle with an LVAD followed by a therapy of different drugs designed to induce myocardial reverse remodelling may contribute to recovery.

It is unknown whether differences in volume unloading of the left ventricle between the continuous-flow rotary pumps and pulsatile pumps may have an impact on myocardial recovery. Similar changes in the degree of cellular recovery between the different pump designs have been observed[138]. Despite a greater degree of volume unloading observed with pulsatile pumps, exercise performance at 3 months after LVAD implantation is similar between the 2 LVAD designs.

The exercise performance after LVAD implantation with a pulsatile, volume displacement pump was not significantly different than exercise performance achieved with a continuous-flow rotary pump with axial design [138].

2.2 Effects on cerebral function and the nervous system

Cerebral blood flow has been shown to correlate with cerebral perfusion pressure over a broad pressure range and showed no significant difference in the response to hypercapnia [139,140]. The effects of an artificial circulation either with pulsatile or non-pulsatile flow on microcirculation in the brain have been monitored and there was no significant difference in blood circulation and metabolism. Other studies suggest there might be some effect on the blood-flow in the brain, these different results may be due to the different experimental conditions [141,142].

Pulsatile flow reperfusion has been shown to be able to improve neurologic outcome. Brain tissue pH, oxygen and carbon dioxide tension as well as cerebral metabolism were demonstrated not be influenced by a non-pulsatile flow [133]. Arterio-jugular venous glucose and lactate differences remained unchanged.

No neural or behavioral abnormalities have been reported [143]. Neurocognitive function was measured before and after operation and there was no difference between continuous and pulsatile VADs. The implantation itself has been shown to improve neurocognitive impairment independently of the type of support.

Ocular circulation was shown to be unchanged as the blood flow in the choroidal microvasculature did not show relevant differences [144].

Peripheral circulatory changes in the auricle suggests capillary autoregulation to maintain appropriate regional blood flow [132,145]. Non pulsatile circulation does not influence vasoactive hormone levels except for a slight increase in norepinephrine. The baroreceptor reflex functions after flow mode conversion.

It has been assumed that pulsatile flow maintained better cerebral blood perfusion and oxygen consumption during reperfusion [142]. There were no significant differences in postoperative electroencephalographic changes and neurocognitive tests among patients who underwent pulsatile versus nonpulsatile support [146]. Pulsatile flow does not seem to be superior to the nonpulsatile perfusion technique. Carotid blood flow showed that the cerebral autoregulation was sufficiently maintained [147-149]. Cerebral oxygen metabolism was not changed by continuous-flow [133]. No significant changes in the carotid blood flow response to hypercapnia were noticed.

The autonomic nervous system has an important function in the control of the circulation and may be influenced by continuous flow. Changes in renal sympathetic nervous activity during nonpulsatile circulation in animal experiments have been reported [145].

2.3 Effects on splanchnic organ function and kidney function

It has been demonstrated that gastric mucosal pH is more reduced with pulseless flow and that splanchnic blood flow is better preserved with pulsatile perfusion [150]. Gastric mucosal tonometry was used to determine the adequacy of the gastrointestinal perfusion. The cardiopulmonary bypass using nonpulsatile flow was associated with the development of gastric mucosal acidosis. Liver and renal functions remained within normal limits.

Coronary artery disease is associated with changes in renal vasculature and chronic renal failure [151]. This study reports that 15% of patients undergoing coronary angiography for coronary artery disease had significant atherosclerotic renovascular disease. Consequently increasing attention is given to avoid a further decrease in renal perfusion during LVAD support. Morphological changes of the arterial systems of the kidneys under prolonged continuous flow left heart bypass are known as a thickening of the media of the afferent arterioles by an increase in the number of smooth muscle cells. Juxtaglomerular areas were expanded and the percentage of anti-proliferating cells was significantly higher thus indicating active proliferation. It appears that continuous-flow support provides adequate renal and hepatic perfusion comparable to that provided by pulsatile support.

Some studies reported effects of non-pulsatile flow on microcirculation and showed differences in renal-arterial and renal-cortical flows associated with pathologic findings in the kidneys in the non-pulsatile group [152,153].
The renal cortex blood flow in the pulsatile group did improve but not in the non-pulsatile group. This suggests that pulsatile assist may be more effective than nonpulsatile in rebuilding the microcirculation after cardiogenic shock. Changes in major organ microcirculations during circulatory support using pulsatile and nonpulsatile pumps suggest that pulsatile assist may improve deteriorated splanchnic organs better than nonpulsatile under the circumstances of acute cardiac shock.

An expansion of the proximal tubes and an expansion of blood capillaries within the glomerulus has been described. A minor decrease in kidney function was observed by other authors [154] but anyway none of the surviving patients needed hemodialysis; one patient in this study required a short period of peritoneal dialysis. Hemolysis or platelet dysfunction was not a clinical problem.

Renal recovery after ischemia is similar with pulsatile and nonpulsatile perfusion when physiological perfusion pressure is achieved [155]. After reperfusion, renal blood flow, oxygen consumption and urine output showed no difference. The histopathologic examination did not differ significantly between the groups. These results suggest that a pulseless pump is acceptable as an assist device as long as a normal flow or perfusion pressure is maintained.
Some studies have reported changes in renal sympathetic nervous activity during nonpulsatile circulation [145]. The creatinine clearance was maintained within the normal range[156].

2.4 Effects on pulmonary function

Studies of continuous-flow show that nonpulsatile circulation may lead to an elevated mean pulmonary artery pressure and higher pulmonary vascular resistance as well as a greater risk for pulmonary edema [157,158]. Arterial and venous occlusion pressure profiles have been measured and during both types of perfusion the occlusion pressure curves were similar. It is not known how the mode of flow changes the resistance in the pulmonary circulation. Perfusion decreases independently of the used flow the pulmonary vascular resistance. This decrease is assumed to be greater for pulsatile than for non-pulsatile flow perfusion.

Other studies about pulmonary arterial pressure and pulmonary vascular resistance between pulsatile and non-pulsatile flows showed no difference with similar blood-gas data [159]. No significant change was observed in either mean pulmonary arterial pressure or pulmonary vascular resistance index between pulsatile and non-pulsatile pumping. There was also no significant change in the ventral to dorsal blood perfusion ratio. These results indicate that pulmonary perfusion functions are not affected by nonpulsatile pulmonary circulation.

Other studies suggested that non-pulsatility may lead to a deterioration of flow distribution [160]. Pulmonary microcirculation was analyzed by vital microscopic observation. Flow distribution during non pulsatile perfusion was heterogeneous compared with pulsatile perfusion.

Pulmonary hypertension was shown to be improved under continuous flow assistance [102,103]. Fixed pulmonary hypertension is a contraindication for cardiac transplantation because of the risk of donor heart failure. The authors could show that left ventricular assist devices decrease fixed pulmonary hypertension and can overcome a contraindication for cardiac transplantation. They conclude that left ventricular assist devices should be considered in all cardiac transplant candidates with fixed pulmonary hypertension. As the post-transplant survival of these patients is uncertain as pulmonary hypertension may reappear, another study showed that long-term post-transplant survival is comparable to cardiac transplant recipients without pulmonary hypertension. It has been demonstrated that elevated pulmonary resistance decreased to normal values during support [102,103,161,162].

Pulmonary oxygen transfer has been shown to be similar with pulsatile and nonpulsatile perfusion [163]. In lung edema pulsatile blood flow was more efficient. No significant changes in gas exchange or intrapulmonary shunt ratio have been observed [164]. This study concludes that pulsatile perfusion during open heart surgical procedure has no advantages in regard to lung water content. The effect of different levels of continuous flow on serum lactate concentration showed an increase at lower perfusion rates [147-149].

The effect of treatmill exercise has been investigated in animals during non-pulsatile support and a decrease of systemic vascular resistance during exercise was observed. Oxygen uptake appears to be less efficient at systemic continuous low flow but there is no difference when the flow is increased [123]. This suggests that flow might be more important than the pulsation in the systemic circulation.

2.5 Effects on endocrine function

The response of vasoactive hormones to flow conversion from pulsatile to non pulsatile mode and vice versa have been assessed and no significant difference was observed neither in blood flow nor in systemic vascular resistance. Different vasoactive hormones have been evaluated and only norepinephrine showed a significant difference between the modes. It has been concluded that non pulsatile perfusion does not influence vasoactive hormone levels in a significant manner except for a slight increase in norepinephrine. The baroreceptor reflex functions in an acute phase after flow mode conversion [132,145].

Neuroendocrine function showed no changes in its circadian rhythm during pulsatile and non-pulsatile left heart assistence [165]. Pulsatile blood flow has been assumed to be of importance for the regulation of endocrine organs. Administration of the hypothalamic releasing hormones revealed normal responses of all pituitary hormones (adrenocorticotropic hormone, thyroid-stimulating hormone, luteinizing hormone and prolactin) except for growth hormone so no major effect on the hypothalamic-pituitary-endorgan system could be demonstrated.

2.6 Outcome

Data from Muenster, Germany showed that cardiac assist devices with continuous flow pattern have similar rates of pre- and posttransplant mortality in comparison with pulsatile LVADs. In this study the rate and severity of posttransplant rejection was higher in the group with continuous flow devices [94]. A study from Italy demonstrated the effectiveness of LVAD therapy in bridging patients with end-stage heart failure to transplantation with good survival rates [166]. Long-term implantable continuous axial-flow pumps have been compared with pulsatile devices. Successful bridging to transplantation and mortality (33.3% vs 36.6%) was similar in both groups [167].

Recent data from UK showed that quality of life appeared to be better in patients with an bridge-to-recovery indication than in bridge to transplantation an heart transplant patients [168].

A prospective, multicenter clinical trial from Australia reported a success rate of 82% (39.4% transplanted, 42.4% transplant-eligible) for the use of the VentrAssist LVAD [82,169].

The US National Circulatory Support Registry showed no difference in clinical outcomes between patients supported with pulsatile and nonpulsatile devices [170]. The rates of weaning and discharge in this study were statistically different and favored patients with univentricular support. Results were the same whether nonpulsatile centrifugal or pulsatile pneumatic devices were used. Although complications were frequent it was rather the patient variables including the age to affect the outcome. One study concludes that pulsatility was more effective than continuous flow in maintaining the perfusion of the microcirculation in end organs after acute shock [152].

Survival after heart transplantation has improved significantly over the last decades. Survival rates at 1, 3, 5 and 7 years after primary cardiac transplantation were 83, 78, 72 and 64% vs 53, 50, 47 and 36%, respectively in retranslantation patients [171]. In 1992 a 5-year-survival rate of over 60% [41] compared to a conservative therapy of patients in the NYHA-stadium IV with a survival rate of only 20-30% in a 2-years-period [172,173] has been reported. More recently a 42% moratlity rate in NYHA classes III and IV has been described [28]. Major causes of death were acute and chronic rejection, infection and sepsis.

Although conservative methods of treatment have constantly been improved 20-30% of the patients listed for transplant die before a suitable donor organ can be assigned to them [174]. At least in the United States heart donor availability has increasingly failed to keep pace with rising demand. Transplant data obtained from the United Network for Organ Sharing showed that a high number of patients died or have been removed from the list each year. Only 49% of patients on the heart transplant waiting list at some time in 1988 underwent the procedure in that year. The major causes of death among waiting patients were congestive heart failure and arrhythmias. The number and proportion of potential recipients who die awaiting heart transplantation is increasing every year. The waiting time may vary from days to several months depending on organ availability, blood group and severity of the disease. Some patients may have serious events such as stroke, infections or kidney failure while waiting for a heart transplant [175].

Data obtained from the National Transplant Database in the UK have been analyzed with a significant difference in the proportions of patients among the different blood groups. Blood group A and AB patients were generally transplanted sooner than O and B patients, with median waiting times of 81 days and 76 days versus 214 days and 174 days respectively. The difference was at least partly due to a large proportion of blood group O hearts being used for non-O patients [176].

The development in the last years showed the possibility of implanting a left ventricular assist device instead of a heart transplant. In this regard a permanent implantation or a temporary mechanical cardiovascular support for full relief of the heart is intended, which allows in selected cases the explantation of the assist device after the recovery of the myocardial function [90,101]. The permanent implantation of a left ventricular assist device would make an immune suppression indispensable and the infection problems and complications arising through acute or chronic rejections, which are associated to transplants, would not occur.

The initial concerns that the contra-physiological, almost non-pulsatile or low-pulsatile flow would have a negative influence on the organ function of the patient has not been confirmed up to now [59,60,161].

The influence of age on outcomes after left ventricular assist device has been studied and it was shown that in the absence of other high risk factors age is no contraindication for LVAD implantation [177].

In general the survival of patients treated by mechanical circulatory support seems to depend more on the underlying condition of the patient than on the type of the assist device. Patients benefit patients through improved survival, functional status and quality of life when compared with inotropic agents, optimum care, or no care. There is little evidence to discriminate between the different device manufacturers.

3. Own Results

3.1 Coronary hemodynamics and myocardial oxygen consumption during support with rotary blood pumps

Peter Voitl MD[1], Michael Vollkron PhD[2,4], Helga Bergmeister DVM[3,4], Georg Wieselthaler MD[2,4], Heinrich Schima PhD[1,2,4]

Artificial Organs 2009; 33(1):77-80

[1]Center for Biomedical Engineering and Physics,
[2]Department for Cardiothoracic Surgery,
[3] Center for Biomedical Research, Med. Univ. of Vienna, Austria;
[4]Ludwig Boltzmann-Cluster for Cardiovascular Research,
Vienna, Austria

3.1.1 Abstract

Mechanical support offered by rotary pumps is increasingly used to assist the failing heart although several questions concerning physiology are remaining. In this study we sought to evaluate the effect of left ventricular assist device therapy on coronary hemodynamics, myocardial oxygen consumption and pulmonary blood flow in sheep. We performed an acute experiment in 10 sheep to obtain invasively measured coronary perfusion data as well as pressure and flow conditions under cardiovascular assistance. A DeBakey VAD® was implanted and systemic and coronary hemodynamic measurements were performed at defined baseline conditions and at five levels of assistance.

Data were measured when the pump was clamped as well as under minimum, maximum and moderate level of assistance, and in a pump-off condition, where backflow occurs.

Coronary flow at the different levels of support showed no significant impact of pump activity. The change from baseline ranged from -10.8 % + 4.6 % (n.s.). In the pulmonary artery we observed a consistent increase in flow up to + 4.5% (n.s.) and a decrease in the pulmonary artery pressure down to − 14.4% (p=0,004). Myocardial oxygen consumption fell with increasing pump support down to -34.6% (P=0,008). Left-ventricular pressure fell about 52.2% (p=0,016) as support was increased.

These results show that blood flow in the coronary arteries is not affected by flow changes imposed by rotary blood pumps. An undiminished coronary perfusion at falling oxygen consumption might contribute to cardiac recovery.

Keywords: Left ventricular assist device—Rotary blood pump — Coronary circulation — animals — oxygen consumption

3.1.2 Introduction

The prevalence of cardiovascular disease is on the increase and currently the most frequent cause of death. For many patients with advanced heart failure, the final treatment option is heart transplantation. However, donor hearts are scarce and frequently unavailable when required. Implantable cardiac support systems allow some of these patients to live and experience an acceptable quality of life over a long period of time. The spectrum of application of these systems is changing as technical improvements are being made and miniature systems are produced. Some of the systems are specifically designed as destination therapy [52,178].

The use of rotary blood pumps has gained widespread acceptance. Rotary blood pumps are small and clinically applicable systems capable of long term support. They are well-suited as an interim therapy for left-ventricular insufficiency as well as an end-stage treatment for patients who cannot undergo transplantation for a variety of reasons [179,180]. Over the last few years these systems have emerged as a feasible alternative to conventional pulsatile pumps, although several questions concerning physiology are still being addressed in a number of studies [60,181-184], including computer models [185]. Aspects of the hemodynamic basis of ventricular assist devices have been discussed particularly with respect to arterial blood flow pulsatility and histologic changes. The effects of rotary blood pumps on coronary blood flow have not been adequately documented; one study showed a decrease in the coronary flow in pigs, with and without a surgically created coronary stenosis [186]. Improved perfusion has been previously registered with the use of pulsatile pump systems [129]. New Information about coronary perfusion and myocardial oxygen consumption is needed to design strategies for optimal unloading and/or training of the heart and to model coronary perfusion during cardiac assist. The purpose of the present study was to investigate the effect of pump flows on coronary parameters in sheep with implanted left-ventricular assist device (DeBakey VAD®).

VAD	Ventricular Assist Device	CVP	Central Venous Pressure
HR	Heart Rate	MVO2	Myocardial oxygen consumption
bpm	Beats per Minute	GUI	Graphical User Interface
LVP	Left Ventricular Pressure	QPulm	Pulmonary artery flow

Table 1: List of abbreviations

3.1.3. Methods

We performed an in vivo investigation during an acute experiment in 10 sheep to determine invasively measured coronary perfusion data as well as pressure and flow conditions under cardiovascular assistance by means of rotary blood pump support of the beating heart. Ten sheep (96+-19 kg) were anesthetized with isoflourane, fentanyl and propofol. A left-sided thoracotomy with resection of the 5th rib was performed and a DeBakey VAD® was implanted between the apex of the left ventricle and the descending aorta. The specific cannulation technique used in these experiments restricts the results to this type of cannulation and VADs connected to the ascending aorta might have a different impact on vascular hemodynamics. An external pacemaker (atrial and ventricular) was used to fix the heart rate and central venous pressure. The study protocol was approved by the ethics committee of the Medical University of Vienna.

Within these ten acute animal experiments 51 hours of data were recorded. The program for data acquisition was developed in Matlab/Simulink and was implemented with a dSpace DS1103 board. The analog input channels had a resolution of 16 bits and the sampling rate was 100 Hz. For each of the baseline conditions shown in table 2, up to five levels of assistance were tested. First, the pump was clamped (simulating no pump), then minimum, maximum and moderate level of assistance were applied and finally a pump-off condition, where backflow occurs, was imposed. The amount of backflow in the pump-off condition was 1.5 to 2 liters per minute.

As it is very difficult to establish a stable model of heart failure, different baseline settings were used to assure identical starting points for the data collection. When the natural heart rate exceeded the fixed pacemaker rate a certain degree of variation of the heart rate or the central venous pressure did occur. The pre-defined baseline conditions for the measurement were the following settings:

1a: CVP = 10 mmHg; HR = 100 bpm
1b: CVP = 10 mmHg; HR = 110 bpm
1c: CVP = 10 mmHg; HR = 130 bpm
1d: CVP = 15 mmHg; HR = 100 bpm
1e: CVP = 15 mmHg; HR = 130 bpm

Table 2: Predefined baseline conditions

Blood samples were taken from central-venous and arterial catheters, and also from a catheter in the coronary sinus which was implanted through the azygous vein. Systemic and coronary hemodynamic measurements were performed at the baseline conditions defined in Table 2. Due to the poor general condition of some sheep, data could not be elicited at all steps in all sheep.

3.1.4 Results

Coronary flow at the different levels of support showed no significant impact of pump activity on the measured flow values in the coronary arteries. Coronary blood flow hardly changed at the different levels of left-ventricular support. As shown in Figure 1, coronary flow was largely unaffected by the various baseline conditions for central venous pressure and heart rate. Data from the moderate level of assistance have been excluded in the figures since these measurements could not be obtained in all animals. The flow in the pulmonary artery showed a constant increase.

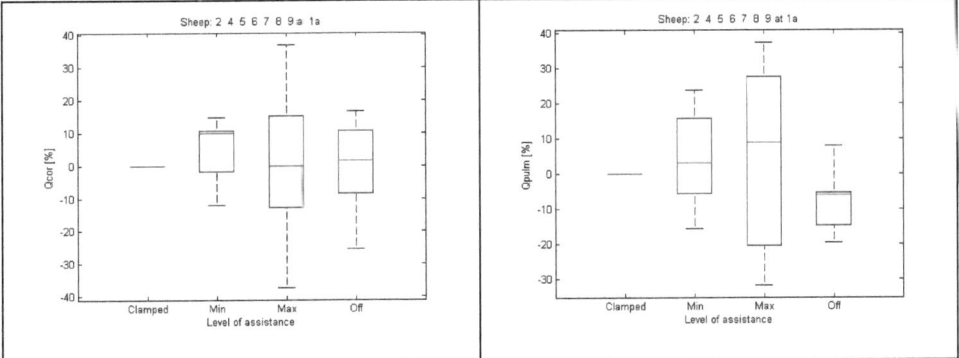

Fig. 1: Coronary blood flow (left) and Pulmonary artery flow (right) at various pump settings, changes from baseline at level 1a: CVP = 10 mmHg; HF = 100 bpm

Myocardial oxygen consumption MVO2 fell as expected with increasing levels of pump support. Both left-ventricular pressure and left atrial pressure decreased as support was increased, suggesting that wall tension was reduced.

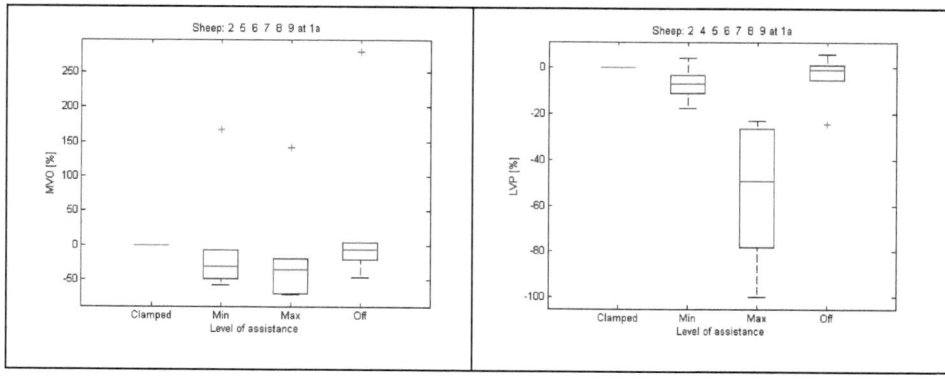

Fig. 2: Myocardial oxygen consumption (left) and left ventricular pressure (right), changes from baseline at level 1a: CVP=10 mmHg; HF=100 bpm

3.1.5 Discussion

Cardiac support systems are implanted essentially for two reasons: on the one hand to ensure sufficient blood pressure and organ perfusion, and on the other hand to reduce the load on the left ventricle and allow the heart to recover [52,184].

It has been shown that an ischemic area can be reduced by improved myocardial blood flow [187]. Furthermore, it has been suspected that one of the major effects of a pump on coronary hemodynamics is the reduction of ventricular load in combination with reduced oxygen consumption [188]. Finally it has been observed that pulmonary hypertension in cardiac transplant candidates can be lowered using left ventricular assist devices [102,103].

In fact very few data are available to show the effect of these pump systems on perfusion parameters in the coronary arteries. Such information is especially important to devise strategies to determine pump settings that optimize perfusion conditions in the left ventricle.

The present experiment showed that blood flow in the coronary arteries is not affected by changes in pump flow, whereas the myocardial oxygen consumption can be reduced by increased levels of mechanical assistance. Alterations in myocardial vascular pressure resulting from changes in myocardial wall tension might be compensated by autoregulatory mechanisms although that was not documented in this series, possibly due to changes in endocardial elasticity secondary to reduced left-ventricular volume under pump support [183].

Falling myocardial oxygen consumption might be explained by the reduced wall tension during enhanced assistance, but constant coronary perfusion could be explained by increased diastolic perfusion pressure. Given the elevated mean pressure and diastolic pressure in the aorta during support, the second effect may possibly act as an additional factor in this setting. Finally, one notes that unaltered coronary perfusion at falling oxygen consumption might contribute significantly to cardiac recovery.

The measured systemic responses at the different settings (table 1) show that the pump reduces the load on the left ventricle and is fully capable of maintaining mean aortic pressure. Furthermore a decreased left-ventricular pressure was observed with increasing pump support.

By nature, changes in the pulmonary artery reflect enhanced LVAD support with increasing flow and reduced pressure. However, this may also be interpreted as a drop in pulmonary vascular resistance: an effect that can help stabilize the right ventricle.

These results reflect, on the one hand, the known hemodynamic effects of rotary blood pumps on pressure conditions in the heart and the large vessels, and signal, on the other hand, the reduced oxygen consumption of the myocardium. The results could be indicative of cardiac recovery. No effect on myocardial flow was registered in the present experiment. The reduced left atrial pressure and increased pulmonary flow that was observed might be indicative of decreased vascular resistance. The pressure-flow relationship of the coronary arteries showed no evidence of an autoregulatory effect.

The limitations of the study are the frequent alterations of pump support and the absence of previous left-heart failure. Investigations of myocardial flow itself would be desirable. Likewise, further studies in hearts with chronic left-heart failure should be performed. A further limitation of the present study is the small number of sheep used and the diverse baseline conditions of the animals. Nevertheless, homogeneous data were obtained within the individual animals.

3.1.6 Conclusion

This study shows, in the acute experiments, that mean coronary flow does not necessarily correlate with changes in pump flows imposed by rotary blood pumps. Unaltered coronary perfusion at falling oxygen consumption during ventricular unloading was observed and might contribute to cardiac recovery.

Acknowledgement

We thank Edward Leonard from the Department of Chemical Engineering, Columbia University, New York, NY, USA for his cooperation and especially for his advice.

3.2 Suction events during left ventricular support and ventricular arrhythmias

Michael Vollkron PhD[2,3], Peter Voitl MD[1], Julia Ta[1], Georg Wieselthaler MD[2,3], Heinrich Schima PhD[1,2,3]

J Heart Lung Transplant 2007;**26**(8):819-25.

[1]Center for Biomedical Engineering and Physics, [2]Department for Cardiothoracic Surgery, Med. Univ. of Vienna, Austria;
[3]Ludwig Boltzmann-Cluster for Cardiovascular Research, Vienna, Austria

3.2.1 Abstract

Background: Axial blood pumps have very successfully entered the arena of prolonged clinical support. However, they do not offer limited inherent load-responsive mechanisms for adjusting pumping performance to venous return and changes in physiological requirements of the patient. Therefore excessive ventricular unloading can be observed in various situations of temporarily reduced venous return. In this study we report severe ventricular arrhythmias closely related to suction events in rotary blood pumps, a phenomenon that has not been described before.

Methods: Data from a clinical trial intended to prove the feasibility of an automatic speed control system for pump recipients were analyzed regarding changes of the electrocardiogram during ventricular collapse. The occurrence of excessive unloading was detected by an automatic suction detection system. The electrocardiagramms were classified semi-manually aided be a graphical user interface. For the statistical analysis of the data a Wilcoxon signed rank test was performed.

Results: Following the automatic suction detection a significant increase of monomorphic ventricular tachycardia from 0.015 to 0.099 events per second ($p<0.05$) was observed. Furthermore it was found that the arrhythmic activity in terms of morphologic ventricular tachycardia did increase after suction from 0.009 to 0.014 events per second.

Conclusion: Excessive ventricular unloading of the left ventricle during continuous left ventricular support can induce ventricular arrhythmias; there is also evidence for an increase of arrhythmic activity after suction. This turned out to be a transient effect which vanishes within five minutes after suction. The ECG-events related to suction have a sudden onset and are severe ventricular arrhythmias, which can consist of even just one extrasystolic beat and they usually cease after clearance of suction.

3.2.2 Introduction

In recent years, fully implantable rotary blood pumps have been used in increasing numbers and have proved to be effective tools for extended cardiac support [189-193]. Most of these devices are used in a constant speed mode, which offers only limited sensitivity (some intrinsic flow increase can be observed with increasing preload and a constant pump speed). Clinical experience has shown that most recipients can be managed by using the contractile reserve of the left ventricle, which acts as a pressure-loading system responsive to changes in venous return [161,193]. A direct adaptation of pump performance to changing demands during exercise, circadian rhythm and different metabolic activities would be highly desirable.

Therefore several systems were recently developed with automatic adaptation to venous return [194-196] and clinical trials are ongoing with devices like the Incor from BerlinHeart and Arrow International, Inc. with CorAide™. The aim of these systems is to react to the changing perfusion demand of the patients by automatic adjustment of pump speed and, a more effective unloading of the ventricle becomes possible. A remaining risk then is that transient changes in venous return can cause excessive unloading of the ventricle. Currently the potential effects of excessive ventricular unloading are not well investigated. Therefore purpose of this study is to gain a better understanding of arrhythmic events in patients under mechanical left ventricular assistance.

We have limited information about the prevalence and clinical significance of suction-induced post-LVAD ventricular arrhythmias. Arrhythmia is defined as a change from the normal rate or control of the heart's contractions, the QRS complex is wide and repolarisation pathways are also different, causing the T wave to have an unusual morphology. It may reduce cardiac output and increase the work of the heart, causing it to require more oxygen.

Although ventricular tachyarrhythmias were common in the basic heart activity of our population a further reduction of complications would be beneficial.

The clinical experience in our center is that excessive unloading can reduce pump flow, increase hemolysis and there are a few cases where patients reported pain during such episodes. Therefore we initiated this retrospective data analysis to investigate the influence of such events on the electrocardiogram. The data used for this study are from the first clinical trial with an automatic speed adaptation system [195] for the DeBakey VAD®. It turned out that patients who experienced partial or complete ventricular collapse during periods of reduced venous return also developed tachyarrhythmia. It was observed that these events usually have a sudden onset and vanish immediately after clearance of excessive ventricular unloading. Similar effects were found in-vivo induced by myocardial contusion in rabbit hearts [197], as well as for patients with pulsatile blood pump support [198].

3.2.3 Methods

DeBakey VAD®: The Pump System includes the titanium pump and inlet cannula, the percutaneous cable, an implantable flow probe, and the outflow graft. It is an axial flow pump of the second generation with mechanical bearings. The components are fully enclosed in a titanium flow tube that has been hermetically sealed. The pump is driven by a brushless, (DC) motor stator that is contained in the stator housing. The pump is attached to a titanium inlet cannula that is placed into the left ventricle. A graft is connected to the pump outlet and anastomosed to the aorta. The positioning of the inflow cannula is very important to avoid any artificial occlusion of the orifice, therefore the inflow cannula was placed parallel to the septum where no inflow reduction by papillary muscles or the lateral wall can occure [199].

Clinical Trial: 19 patients participated in a first clinical study with the aim to investigate the feasibility of an automatic speed control system for the DeBakey VAD®. These pump recipients were tested in 57 sessions and an overall number of 105.5 hours of data were recorded. To capture a broad spectrum of patient conditions, activities from different clinical settings were evaluated. Postoperatively, tests were performed under stationary conditions and during common intensive care maneuvers. On standard ward, simulations of everyday life took place. After initial recovery, patients in the standard ward and also after discharge from the hospital were investigated in sessions lasting as long as three hours. These tests included lying, sitting, repeated bicycling exercise, eating, drinking, coughing and valsalva maneuvers. Finally, five patients underwent micro-catheter evaluation anticipating transplantation. They were studied while fully monitored spiroergometry was performed. Because of the invasiveness of this procedure, it was only performed as part of a procedure required for the patients' transplantation. Within this setting, the patient underwent two standardized bicycle-ergometry runs involving a power increase of 25 watts for 5 minutes.

ECG: The rhythm strip of the electrocardiogram was monitored by the use of a clinical Horizon-Monitor (Mennen Medical Ltd. Model 260) equipped with an analog output interface. This analog signal was recorded with a dSpace® DS1103 board at a sampling rate of 100 Hz. As no 12-lead ECG has been used, the electrocardiography site of origin of the ventricular tachycardia has not been identified.

Suction Detection: The developed suction detection system is based on the observation of the measured pump flow signal in the time domain. It provides a continuous analysis of the flow pattern regarding the appearance of seven individual indicators for excessive ventricular unloading within each heart cycle. Please find a list of these indicators in the following, for details please refer to [108]:

1. The *Asymmetry Criteria* compares the maximum slew rate of the falling edge of the pump flow with the maximum slew rate of the consecutive rising edge.
2. The *Plateau Criteria* checks the pump flow signal for significant flow reductions after periods of constant (non-pulsatile) blood flow.
3. The *Slew Rate Criteria* calculates the slew rate of the falling edge of the pulsatile pump flow signal and compares it to a constant threshold level.
4. The *Low Flow Criteria* indicates cases of complete ventricular collapses by detection of prolonged periods of zero pump flow without backflow condition.
5. The *Mean-Min-Max Criteria* determines the difference between the amplitudes of the mean flow value to the minimum respectively maximum flow value.
6. The *Saddle-Neg Criteria* is characterized by saddle formations in the falling arch of the flow peak.
7. The *Saddle-Pos Criteria* indicates suction in case of saddle formations on the rising arch of the flow peak.

From comparison with ultrasound measurements in pump recipients it is known that this system is capable of detecting not only complete but also partial collapse of the left ventricle. A more detailed description regarding this automatic suction detection system are previously published [109,194].

Classification of changes in the rhythm strip QRS morphology: The classification of the ECG data has been done manually. For efficient classification a graphical user interface was developed in Matlab which offers quick access to the continuous data record as well as easy selection and scoring for the individual events. The observed events were grouped into the following categories (see figure 1a):

- Type 1: Single ventricular extra systolic event (SVE)
- Type 2: Monomorphic ventricular tachycardia (MVT) - The QRS complexes within an episode of tachycardia do not change the morphology from one beat to the next, sometimes called "univocal"
- Type 3: Polymorphic ventricular tachycardia (PVT) - Series of different pathologic QRS complexes not meeting the criteria for MVT
- Type 4: Ventricular fibrillation (VF) - A ventricular arrhythmia consisting of a fibrillating and highly irregular activity with no identifiable QRS shape.
- Type 5: Unclassifiable - No basic rhythmologic pattern was observable
- Type 6: Uncertain (for later discussion) – These patterns were analyzed in detail after a first classification process

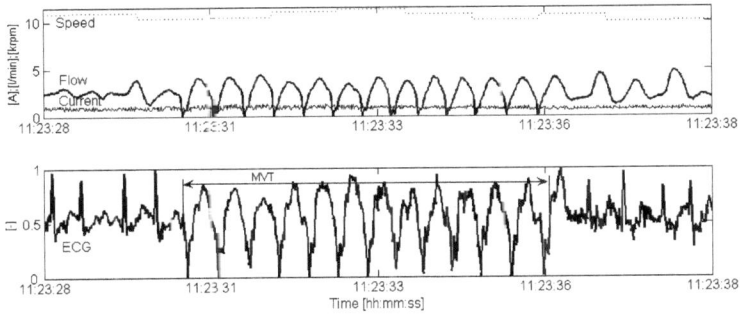

Figure 1: Series of monomorphic ventricular tachycardia beats induced by excessive ventricular unloading.

Arrhythmias were considered as severe when they were grade 1 or more in the Lowns classification of arrhythmias regardless of their clinical value. Thus supraventricular and minor arrhythmias were not included.

Statistics: For statistical analysis the mean values of arrhythmias/sec were paired for each patient and analyzed in a Wilcoxon signed rank test.

Patients: The clinical study was done in full compliance with the Helsinki declaration and approved by the Ethics Board of the University with a written informed consent form signed by each patient. The basic cardiac arrhythmias as well as the changes during suction events have been recorded, regardless of the underlying medication or the basic heart condition.

3.2.4 Results

From the nineteen patients included in this study, four never developed any detected suction events during the test. Therefore these four patients were excluded from this retrospective study. Figure 1 shows a typical example for a MVT triggered by excessive ventricular unloading.

The basic arrhythmic activity of the individual patients is given in figure 2.

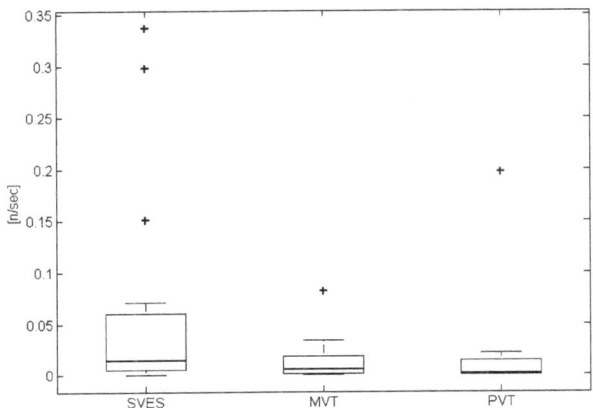

Figure 2: Description of the basic arrhythmic activity of 19 DeBakey VAD recipients using a box plot. The crosses show the outliers which represents values that are more that 1.5 times the interquartile range away from the top of the box. Four of those patients did not experience any suction and two of them did not develop any arrhythmic events.

	SVES	MVT	PVT	VF	Σ
#	4009	912	336	16	5273
Duration [sec]	2596	2262	607	77	5542

Table1:
Summary of all classified arrhythmic events and their duration.

Ventricular fibrillation was rarely observed (see table 1) and never related to suction detection and therefore excluded. Particular examples for SVES, MVT and PVT are given in figure 3. The high standard variation for SVES events is due to the frequent occurrence in three of these patients (0.151, 0.298, 0.337 [n/sec]).

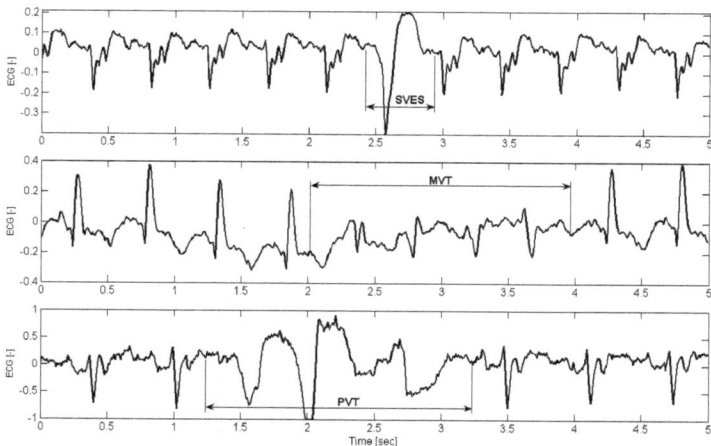

Figure 3:

Examples for the occurrence of SVES, MVT and PVT. The classification was done manually, aided by a graphical userinterface.

Table 2 gives the total number of suction detection, 85% of them are based on the "Plateau" and "MeanMin" criterion. The second row of table 2 gives the duration; in total we observed 0.013 events per second.

	Plateau	LowFlow	SlewRate	Asymmerty	SaddleNeg	SaddlePos	MeanMin	Σ
$^{-3}$	183	2	3	44	25	25	387	669
/sec]	3.74	0.03	0.05	0.83	0.42	0.63	7.64	13.35

Table2:
Summary of the total number of individual suction detections and the suction rate per second.

Table 3 gives the number of suction detections which correlates with arrhythmic events and the percentage with reference to the total number of occurrences.

Comparing the basal arrhythmic activity of each patient to those arrhythmic events situated within a range of ±2 seconds around suction it turned out that the occurrence of MVT (8 patients. 51 events) did increase significantly compared to the baseline activity (see figure 4).

	Plateau	LowFlow	SlewRate	Asymmerty	SaddleNeg	SaddlePos	MeanMin	Σ
#	66	2	3	14	4	5	162	256
[%]	36	100	100	32	16	20	42	38

Table3:
Summary of all suction detections, which correlates with arrhythmic events and their percentage regarding the total amount of detections.

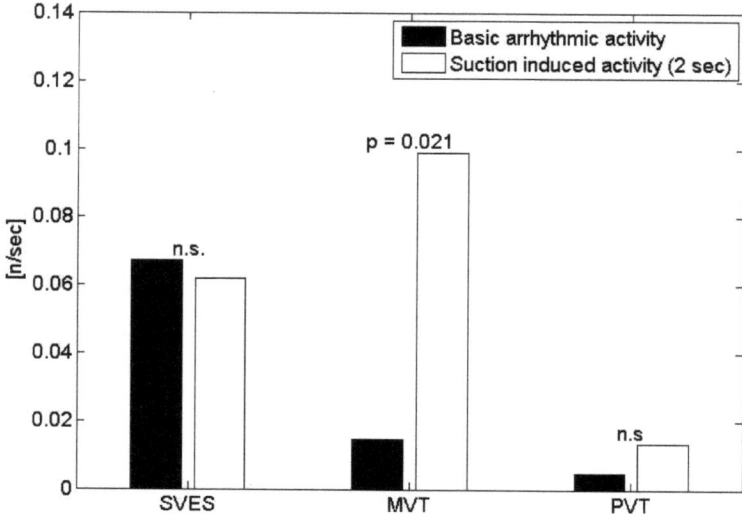

Figure 4:
Comparison of the basic arrhythmic activity with the arrhythmic activity observed within a time window of 2 seconds before, verses after, suction detection.

SVES (9 patients, 20 events) and PVT (3 patients, 9 events) were not significant. To evaluate the arrhythmic events per second within a time window of 2 seconds around suction detection, subsequent suction detections with a delay of less than 4 seconds were collected into groups. The same procedure was applied to evaluate the arrhythmic activity 60 seconds before respectively after single or groups of suction detection. An additional transition period of 5 seconds was placed to avoid the inclusion of suction triggered arrhythmias. In this case consecutive suction detections were grouped if the delay between them was smaller than 65 seconds (60 seconds observation plus 5 seconds transition time).

Figure 5 shows that the comparison of the arrhythmic activity within a time frame of 60 seconds (5 seconds transition period) before, verses after, suction does not lead to statistically significant results.

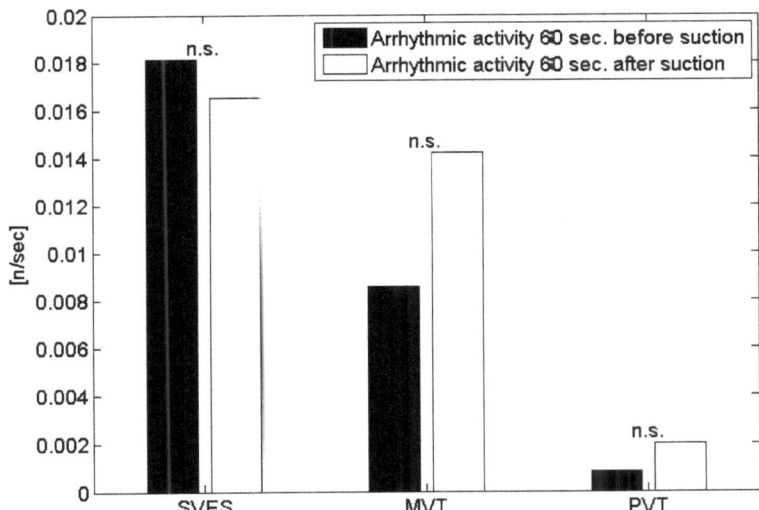

Figure 5:
Comparison of the arrhythmic activity within a time window of 60 seconds (5 seconds transition period) before verses after suction. The results are not significant (Wilcoxon signed rank test) however an increase of MVT can be observed.

However an increase of MVT of 65.12 % before and after suction can be observed. On the other hand the occurrence of SVES and PVT changed only slightly. Figure 6 shows that this effect of increased MVT activity after suction events decays within the following five minutes.

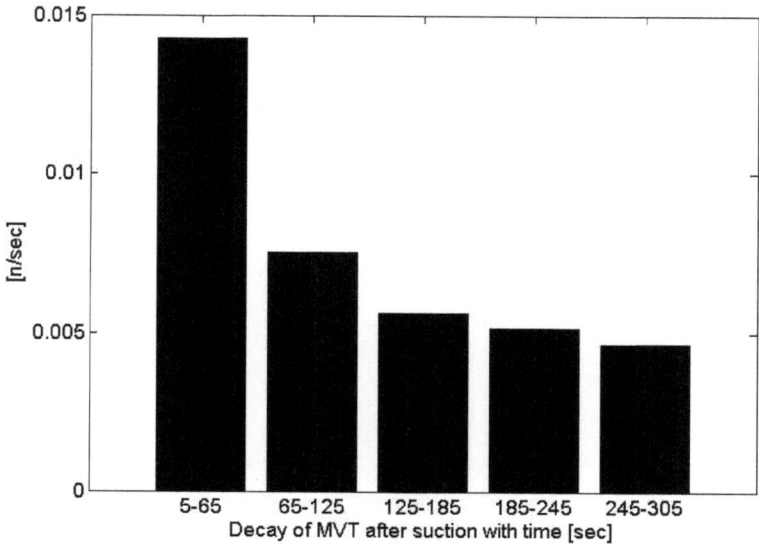

Figure 6:

The amount of MVT events per second observed after suction decreases with time

This observation raises the question if this increased activity is related to the basal arrhythmic activity. To answer this patients are sorted according to basal arrhythmic activity. Figure 7 depicts that those patients whom experienced more frequently (more that 0.05 n/sec, see figure 7 right side) arrhythmic episodes are also those responsible for the increase of MVT's subsequent to suction episodes.

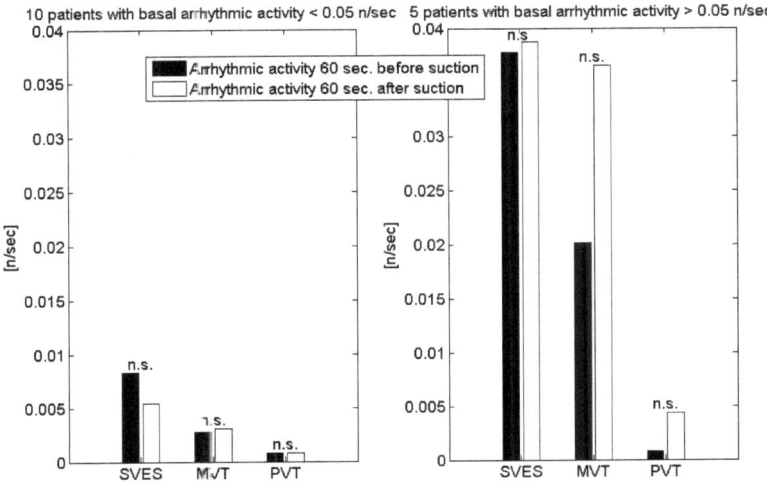

Figure 7:
Comparison of the arrhythmic activity before and after suction episodes of patients with basal activity less that 0.05 n/sec, respectively over 0.05 n/sec. The observation window was chosen to start after a transition period of 5 seconds before respectively after suction.

Finally it was investigated if there is a correlation between the basic arrhythmic activity and the appearance of suction. However from the currently available data set it was not possible to find such a correlation. Possible reasons for that are the skewed data which is represented by the low median value in the box plots given in figure 2, and the wide spread distribution of the basal conditions of the individual patients, both related to the limited number of participants in the study.

3.2.5 Discussion

This study is a systematic approach to investigate the impact of excessive ventricular unloading on the cardiac rhythm of the patient. Several factors that may influence the cardiac rhythm of mechanical cardiac assist recipients are currently in discussion: trauma, especially when the LV collapses and the device surface has direct contact with the endocardium as it is seen when catheters induce arrhythmias; a sensitive zone around the inflow cannula at the apex and electrolyte shift induced by the ventricular unloading as well as a direct traumatizing effect on the heart [197,200-205].

The mechanisms involved in cardiac decompensation and the effects of mechanical unloading of the failing human heart with a continuous-flow pump have been studied with fluorescence labeling and microscopy [206,207]. These specific factors and their changes and the biochemical and mechanical alterations caused by them may contribute to a different sensitivity for heart arrhythmias. Especially the Ca++ metabolism can lead to membrane disruption [208]. The alpha adrenoreceptor (AR) signal system is known to regulate the Ca++ metabolism. After heart failure-induced AR down-regulation, an up-regulation in 1ARs has been described as a result of LVAD unloading [207]. The fact that mechanical unloading of the myocardium is associated with significant changes in 1AR density could have a protective effect against arrhythmias. It has also been observed that under mechanical unloading changes in the levels of cytokine and nitric oxide synthase may lead the heart into a protective and repair mode, this could contribute to an altered susceptibility against arrhythmias as well [206].

For pulsatile devices, a significant increase of extra systolic events has been reported [198]. The immediate correlation with periods of excessive ventricular unloading during non-pulsatile support is not yet known. How ischemia works as a pathogen factor cannot be assessed properly at the current stage.

What was uncovered in this investigation is a statistically significant increase of severe MVT's triggered by suction events (see figure 1) compared to the basal arrhythmic activity occurred regardless of whether this basic activity has been high or low. These arrhythmias have a sudden onset and they usually cease immediately after clearance of suction. This behavior cannot be explained by electrolyte shift due to the reaction time of onset and clearance. It is more likely a reaction to the possible trauma induced by the suction event. On the other hand, the amount of SVES and PVT triggered by suction were not significant but repeatedly observed (SVES: 9 patients, 20 events; PVT: 3 patients, 9 events).

A second observation was that the occurrence of MVT's within a time frame of 60 seconds subsequent to suction episodes increased by 65.12% over the occurrence prior to the suction event. This effect was found not to be statistically significant at least by means of the Wilcoxon signed rank test which we are limited to since we cannot assume a normal distribution in our data set. In figure 6 it can be seen that this effect decays within the following five minutes after suction. This transient, but not persistent arrhythmogenic effect, strengthens the hypothesis that trauma is the cause of the arrhythmias.

Certainly this study has also some inherent limitations: It was done retrospectively on a dataset, which was primarily intended for a clinical study on control algorithms. We did not use a 12 lead ECG since the focus of the original clinical study was to prove the feasibility of an automatic control algorithm for the DeBakey VAD®. Therefore, the ECG record was primarily applied to monitor the heart rate. Although we are aware of the fact that some bias may have been in our ECG interpretations, the mitigating factor for that is that the manual classification was done by a cardiologist who was not involved in this investigation. Because of ethical reasons, suction was not intentionally induced in patients and was avoided by manual reduction of speed in the non-controlled measurement periods or by the automatic control algorithm. The reader must be aware of these censoring effects on the data sets. However, such mediating effects would underscore the basic finding of the study, that suction can cause additional severe short term arrhythmia.

3.2.6 Conclusion

It was shown that excessive ventricular unloading of the left ventricle during continuous left ventricular support can induce arrhythmias. These ventricular arrhythmias related to suction have a sudden onset and usually cease after clearance of suction.

We could show an increase in de novo MVT ($p = 0.021$) during suction events in patients with rotary blood pumps. Furthermore we could observe an increase of MVT of 65% between arrhythmic activity 60 seconds before and after suction. This increase turned out to be a short time effect which vanishes within several minutes following the suction event. In contrary, the incidence of SVES or PVT showed only slight changes.

Additionally, there is evidence of a relationship between increased arrhythmic activity following suction events and basal activity. We conclude that suction events in rotary blood pumps may cause severe ventricular arrhythmias and needs to be avoided, or at least reduced. Whether these post-LVAD ventricular arrhythmias are associated with an adverse clinical outcome needs to be investigated further.

Acknowledgement:

We thank Robert Benkowski and Gino Morello from MicroMed Cardiovascular Inc, Houston, for their cooperation and especially for their adaptation of equipment for data collection.

4. Conclusion

Recent clinical trials have shown that rotary pumps have excellent potential for helping patients to recover from end-stage heart disease and resulting in a good quality of life.

The effects of low pulsatility or even pulseless circulation on the physiology of organ function are not yet fully understood. Our research concerning the effects of rotary blood pumps may contribute to further improvement in the development of monitoring and control techniques of rotary blood pump systems.

5. References

1. Moskowitz AJ, Rose EA, Gelijns AC. The cost of long-term LVAD implantation. *Ann Thorac Surg* 2001;**71**(3 Suppl):S195-8; discussion S203-4.
2. Beyersdorf F. Economics of ventricular assist devices: European view. *Ann Thorac Surg* 2001;**71**(3 Suppl):S192-4; discussion S202-3.
3. Arabia FA, Smith RG, Jaffe C, et al. Cost analysis of the Novacor Left Ventricular Assist System as an outpatient bridge to heart transplantation. *Asaio J* 1996;**42**(5):M546-9.
4. Zannad F, Stough WG, Pitt B, et al. Heart failure as an endpoint in heart failure and non-heart failure cardiovascular clinical trials: the need for a consensus definition. *Eur Heart J* 2008;**29**(3):413-21.
5. Angermayr L. GM, Busse R. Künstliche Ventrikel bei fortgeschrittener Herzinsuffizienz. *Schriftenreihe Health Technology Assessment (HTA) in der Bundesrepublik Deutschland* 2007.
6. Bleumink GS, Knetsch AM, Sturkenboom MC, et al. Quantifying the heart failure epidemic: prevalence, incidence rate, lifetime risk and prognosis of heart failure The Rotterdam Study. *Eur Heart J* 2004;**25**(18):1614-9.
7. Funk M. Epidemiology of end-stage heart disease. In: Hogness JR, Vanantwerp M, eds. The artificial heart: prototypes, policies, and patients. *Washington: National Academic Press* 1991:1991: 251-261.
8. Pearte CA, Furberg CD, O'Meara ES, et al. Characteristics and baseline clinical predictors of future fatal versus nonfatal coronary heart disease events in older adults: the Cardiovascular Health Study. *Circulation* 2006;**113**(18):2177-85.
9. Oosterlee AR, A.; van Zweet, W. Annual Report 2006. *Eurotransplant International Foundation* 2006.
10. Hunt SA, Abraham WT, Chin MH, et al. ACC/AHA 2005 Guideline Update for the Diagnosis and Management of Chronic Heart Failure in the Adult: a report of the American College of Cardiology/American Heart Association Task Force on Practice Guidelines (Writing Committee to Update the 2001 Guidelines for the Evaluation and Management of Heart Failure): developed in collaboration with the American College of Chest Physicians and the International Society for Heart and Lung Transplantation:

endorsed by the Heart Rhythm Society. *Circulation* 2005;**112**(12):e154-235.
11. Rudiger A, Harjola VP, Muller A, et al. Acute heart failure: clinical presentation, one-year mortality and prognostic factors. *Eur J Heart Fail* 2005;**7**(4):662-70.
12. Nieminen MS, Bohm M, M RC, et al. [Executive summary of the guidelines on the diagnosis and treatment of acute heart failure]. *Ital Heart J Suppl* 2005;**6**(4):218-54.
13. Poole-Wilson PA. Differences in European and North American approaches to the management of heart failure. *Cardiol Clin* 2008;**26**(1):107-12, viii.
14. Lund LH, Mancini D. Heart failure in women. *Med Clin North Am* 2004;**88**(5):1321-45, xii.
15. He J, Ogden LG, Bazzano LA, Vupputuri S, Loria C, Whelton PK. Risk factors for congestive heart failure in US men and women: NHANES I epidemiologic follow-up study. *Arch Intern Med* 2001;**161**(7):996-1002.
16. Kardys I, Knetsch AM, Bleumink GS, et al. C-reactive protein and risk of heart failure. The Rotterdam Study. *Am Heart J* 2006;**152**(3):514-20.
17. van Vark LC, Kardys I, Bleumink GS, et al. Lipoprotein-associated phospholipase A2 activity and risk of heart failure: The Rotterdam study. *Eur Heart J* 2006;**27**(19):2346-52.
18. Vitale C, Miceli M, Rosano GM. Gender-specific characteristics of atherosclerosis in menopausal women: risk factors, clinical course and strategies for prevention. *Climacteric* 2007;**10 Suppl 2**:16-20.
19. Kardys I, Deckers JW, Stricker BH, Vletter WB, Hofman A, Witteman JC. Echocardiographic parameters and all-cause mortality: The Rotterdam Study. *Int J Cardiol* 2008.
20. Brignole M, Bellardine Black CL, Bloch Thomsen PE, et al. Improved Arrhythmia Detection in Implantable Loop Recorders. *J Cardiovasc Electrophysiol* 2008.
21. Cleland JG, Coletta AP, Yassin A, et al. Clinical trials update from the American College of Cardiology 2008: CARISMA, TRENDS, meta-analysis of Cox-2 studies, HAT, ON-TARGET, HYVET, ACCOMPLISH, MOMENTUM, PROTECT, HORIZON-HF and REVERSE. *Eur J Heart Fail* 2008.

22. Conroy RM, Pyorala K, Fitzgerald AP, et al. Estimation of ten-year risk of fatal cardiovascular disease in Europe: the SCORE project. *Eur Heart J* 2003;**24**(11):987-1003.
23. Ulmer H, Kollerits B, Kelleher C, Diem G, Concin H. Predictive accuracy of the SCORE risk function for cardiovascular disease in clinical practice: a prospective evaluation of 44 649 Austrian men and women. *Eur J Cardiovasc Prev Rehabil* 2005;**12**(5):433-41.
24. Woodward M, Huxley H, Lam TH, Barzi F, Lawes CM, Ueshima H. A comparison of the associations between risk factors and cardiovascular disease in Asia and Australasia. *Eur J Cardiovasc Prev Rehabil* 2005;**12**(5):484-91.
25. Kannel WB; Savage DC, WP. Cardiac failure in the Framingham study: twentyyear follow-up. *Braunwald E, Mock MB, Watson JT, eds. Congestive heart failure.* New York: Grune & Stratton 1981:15-30.
26. McKee PC, WP: McNamara, PM; Kannel, WB. The natural history of congestive heart failure: the Framingham study. *NEJM* 1971;**285**:1441-1446.
27. Assmann G, Cullen P, Schulte H. Simple scoring scheme for calculating the risk of acute coronary events based on the 10-year follow-up of the prospective cardiovascular Munster (PROCAM) study. *Circulation* 2002;**105**(3):310-5.
28. Ahmed A. A propensity matched study of New York Heart Association class and natural history end points in heart failure. *Am J Cardiol* 2007;**99**(4):549-53.
29. Felker GM, Thompson RE, Hare JM, et al. Underlying causes and long-term survival in patients with initially unexplained cardiomyopathy. *N Engl J Med* 2000;**342**(15):1077-84.
30. Komoda T, Drews T, Lehmkuhl HB, Hetzer R. Role of ventricular assist devices in the German heart allocation system. *J Artif Organs* 2006;**9**(1):29-33.
31. Komoda T, Hetzer R, Lehmkuhl HB. Destiny of candidates for heart transplantation in the Eurotransplant heart allocation system. *Eur J Cardiothorac Surg* 2008.

32. Rose EA, Gelijns AC, Moskowitz AJ, et al. Long-term mechanical left ventricular assistance for end-stage heart failure. *N Engl J Med* 2001;**345**(20):1435-43.
33. Teo KK, Yusuf S, Pfeffer M, et al. Effects of long-term treatment with angiotensin-converting-enzyme inhibitors in the presence or absence of aspirin: a systematic review. *Lancet* 2002;**360**(9339):1037-43.
34. Pfeffer MA. Mechanistic lessons from the SAVE Study. Survival and Ventricular Enlargement. *Am J Hypertens* 1994;**7**(9 Pt 2):106S-111S.
35. Hogness J. Preface. In: Hogness JR, Vanantwerp M, eds. *The artificial heart: prototypes, policies, and patients*. 1991(National Academic Press):i-x.
36. Aronow WS. What is the appropriate treatment of hypertension in elders? *J Gerontol A Biol Sci Med Sci* 2002;**57**(8):M483-6.
37. Aronow WS. Treatment of older persons with hypercholesterolemia with and without cardiovascular disease. *J Gerontol A Biol Sci Med Sci* 2001;**56**(3):M138-45.
38. Aronow WS, Ahn C. Frequency of congestive heart failure in older persons with prior myocardial infarction and serum low-density lipoprotein cholesterol > or = 125 mg/dl treated with statins versus no lipid-lowering drug. *Am J Cardiol* 2002;**90**(2):147-9.
39. Nayak D, Aronow WS. Effect of an ongoing educational program on the use of antiplatelet drugs, beta-blockers, angiotensin-converting enzyme inhibitors, and lipid-lowering drugs in patients with coronary artery disease seen in an academic cardiology clinic. *Cardiol Rev* 2005;**13**(2):95-7.
40. Ghosh S, Aronow WS. Utilization of lipid-lowering drugs in elderly persons with increased serum low-density lipoprotein cholesterol associated with coronary artery disease, symptomatic peripheral arterial disease, prior stroke, or diabetes mellitus before and after an educational program on dyslipidemia treatment. *J Gerontol A Biol Sci Med Sci* 2003;**58**(5):M432-5.
41. Kaye M. The registry of the International Society for Heart and Lung Transplatation:. *Journal of Heart and Lung Transplantation* 1992;**11**(599-606).
42. Young JB, Naftel DC, Bourge RC, et al. Matching the heart donor and heart transplant recipient. Clues for successful expansion of the donor pool: a multivariable, multiinstitutional report. The Cardiac Transplant Research

Database Group. *J Heart Lung Transplant* 1994;**13**(3):353-64; discussion 364-5.
43. Tamisier D, Vouhe P, Le Bidois J, Mauriat P, Khoury W, Leca F. Donor-recipient size matching in pediatric heart transplantation: a word of caution about small grafts. *J Heart Lung Transplant* 1996;**15**(2):190-5.
44. Deng MC, De Meester JM, Smits JM, Heinecke J, Scheld HH. Effect of receiving a heart transplant: analysis of a national cohort entered on to a waiting list, stratified by heart failure severity. Comparative Outcome and Clinical Profiles in Transplantation (COCPIT) Study Group. *Bmj* 2000;**321**(7260):540-5.
45. Copeland JG, 3rd, Smith RG, Arabia FA, et al. Comparison of the CardioWest total artificial heart, the novacor left ventricular assist system and the thoratec ventricular assist system in bridge to transplantation. *Ann Thorac Surg* 2001;**71**(3 Suppl):S92-7; discussion S114-5.
46. Copeland JG, Arabia FA, Tsau PH, et al. Total artificial hearts: bridge to transplantation. *Cardiol Clin* 2003;**21**(1):101-13.
47. El-Banayosy A, Korfer R, Arusoglu L, et al. Device and patient management in a bridge-to-transplant setting. *Ann Thorac Surg* 2001;**71**(3 Suppl):S98-102; discussion S114-5.
48. El-Banayosy A, Arusoglu L, Morshuis M, et al. CardioWest total artificial heart: Bad Oeynhausen experience. *Ann Thorac Surg* 2005;**80**(2):548-52.
49. Sun BC. Indications for long-term assist device placement as bridge to transplantation. *Cardiol Clin* 2003;**21**(1):51-5.
50. Samuels LE, Dowling R. Total artificial heart: destination therapy. *Cardiol Clin* 2003;**21**(1):115-8.
51. Tsukui H, Teuteberg JJ, Murali S, et al. Biventricular assist device utilization for patients with morbid congestive heart failure: a justifiable strategy. *Circulation* 2005;**112**(9 Suppl):I65-72.
52. Westaby S. Ventricular assist devices as destination therapy. *Surg Clin North Am* 2004;**84**(1):91-123.
53. Nwaejike N, Bonde P, Campalani G. Complete mechanical circulatory support using ventricular assist devices for post-cardiotomy biventricular failure. *Ulster Med J* 2008;**77**(1):36-8.

54. Park SJ, Tector A, Piccioni W, et al. Left ventricular assist devices as destination therapy: a new look at survival. *J Thorac Cardiovasc Surg* 2005;**129**(1):9-17.
55. Moon MR, Castro LJ, DeAnda A, et al. Right ventricular dynamics during left ventricular assistance in closed-chest dogs. *Ann Thorac Surg* 1993;**56**(1):54-66; discussion 66-7.
56. Loebe M, Hennig E, Muller J, Spiegelsberger S, Weng Y, Hetzer R. Long-term mechanical circulatory support as a bridge to transplantation, for recovery from cardiomyopathy, and for permanent replacement. *Eur J Cardiothorac Surg* 1997;**11 Suppl**:S18-24.
57. Liden H, Karason K, Bergh CH, Nilsson F, Koul B, Wiklund L. The feasibility of left ventricular mechanical support as a bridge to cardiac recovery. *Eur J Heart Fail* 2007;**9**(5):525-30.
58. Quaini E, Pavie A, Chieco S, Mambrito B. The Concerted Action 'Heart' European registry of clinical application of mechanical circulatory support systems: bridge to transplant. The Registry Scientific Committee. *Eur J Cardiothorac Surg* 1997;**11**(1):182-8.
59. Saito S, Nishinaka T. Chronic nonpulsatile blood flow is compatible with normal end-organ function: implications for LVAD development. *J Artif Organs* 2005;**8**(3):143-8.
60. Thalmann M, Schima H, Wieselthaler G, Wolner E. Physiology of continuous blood flow in recipients of rotary cardiac assist devices. *J Heart Lung Transplant* 2005;**24**(3):237-45.
61. Wray J, Hallas CN, Banner NR. Quality of life and psychological well-being during and after left ventricular assist device support. *Clin Transplant* 2007;**21**(5):622-7.
62. Lietz K, Long JW, Kfoury AG, et al. Outcomes of left ventricular assist device implantation as destination therapy in the post-REMATCH era: implications for patient selection. *Circulation* 2007;**116**(5):497-505.
63. Reichenbach SH, Farrar DJ, Hill JD. A versatile intracorporeal ventricular assist device based on the thoratec VAD system. *Ann Thorac Surg* 2001;**71**(3 Suppl):S171-5; discussion S183-4.
64. Hetzer R, Loebe M, Potapov EV, et al. Circulatory support with pneumatic paracorporeal ventricular assist device in infants and children. *Ann Thorac Surg* 1998;**66**(5):1498-506.

65. Hetzer R, Loebe M, Weng Y, Alexi-Meskhishvili V, Stiller B. Pulsatile pediatric ventricular assist devices: Current results for bridge to transplantation. *Semin Thorac Cardiovasc Surg Pediatr Card Surg Annu* 1999;**2**:157-176.
66. Stiller B, Dahnert I, Weng YG, Hennig E, Hetzer R, Lange PE. Children may survive severe myocarditis with prolonged use of biventricular assist devices. *Heart* 1999;**82**(2):237-40.
67. Pennington DG, McBride LR, Swartz MT. Implantation technique for the Novacor left ventricular assist system. *J Thorac Cardiovasc Surg* 1994;**108**(4):604-8.
68. Minami K, Knyphausen E, Suzuki R, et al. Mechanical ventricular circulatory support in children; Bad Oeynhausen experience. *Ann Thorac Cardiovasc Surg* 2005;**11**(5):307-12.
69. Saito S, Westaby S, Piggot D, et al. End-organ function during chronic nonpulsatile circulation. *Ann Thorac Surg* 2002;**74**(4):1080-5.
70. Noon GP, Morley DL, Irwin S, Abdelsayed SV, Benkowski RJ, Lynch BE. Clinical experience with the MicroMed DeBakey ventricular assist device. *Ann Thorac Surg* 2001;**71**(3 Suppl):S133-8; discussion S144-6.
71. Noon GP, Morley D, Irwin S, Abdelsayed S, Benkowski R, Lynch BE. Turbine blood pumps. *Adv Card Surg* 2001;**13**:169-91.
72. Wolner E. Leistungsbericht 2006. Vienna: http://www.meduniwien.ac.at/Herz-Thorax-Chirurgie/leistung06.htm, 2006.
73. Vollkron M. Development of an automatic speed adaption system for continuous working left ventricular assist devices. Dissertation: TU Wien, 2004.
74. Hoshi H, Shinshi T, Takatani S. Third-generation blood pumps with mechanical noncontact magnetic bearings. *Artif Organs* 2006;**30**(5):324-38.
75. Tsukui H WS, Stanford E, Teuteberg JL, Kormos RL. Does a rotary pump provide full cardiac decompression and circulatory support? *ASAIO J* 2005;**51(2)**:28A.
76. Frazier OH, Gemmato C, Myers TJ, et al. Initial clinical experience with the HeartMate II axial-flow left ventricular assist device. *Tex Heart Inst J* 2007;**34**(3):275-81.

77. Frazier OH, Delgado RM, 3rd, Kar B, Patel V, Gregoric ID, Myers TJ. First clinical use of the redesigned HeartMate II left ventricular assist system in the United States: a case report. *Tex Heart Inst J* 2004;**31**(2):157-9.
78. Heartware. http://www.heartware.com.au/IRM/content/usa/products_HVAD.html. Framingham, Massachusetts, 2007.
79. Wieselthaler GM, Schima H, Hiesmayr M, et al. First clinical experience with the DeBakey VAD continuous-axial-flow pump for bridge to transplantation. *Circulation* 2000;**101**(4):356-9.
80. Fraser CD, Jr., Carberry KE, Owens WR, et al. Preliminary experience with the MicroMed DeBakey pediatric ventricular assist device. *Semin Thorac Cardiovasc Surg Pediatr Card Surg Annu* 2006:109-14.
81. Morales DL, Dibardino DJ, McKenzie ED, et al. Lessons learned from the first application of the DeBakey VAD Child: an intracorporeal ventricular assist device for children. *J Heart Lung Transplant* 2005;**24**(3):331-7.
82. Esmore DS, Kaye D, Salamonsen R, et al. First clinical implant of the VentrAssist left ventricular assist system as destination therapy for end-stage heart failure. *J Heart Lung Transplant* 2005;**24**(8):1150-4.
83. Boujoukos AJ, Martich GD. Mechanical circulatory assist devices. *J Intensive Care Med* 1996;**11**(1):23-36.
84. Leibundgut G, Brunner-La Rocca HP. End-stage chronic heart failure. *Swiss Med Wkly* 2007;**137**(7-8):107-13.
85. Morgan JA, Stewart AS, Lee BJ, Oz MC, Naka Y. Role of the Abiomed BVS 5000 device for short-term support and bridge to transplantation. *Asaio J* 2004;**50**(4):360-3.
86. Hetzer R, Hennig E, Schiessler A, Friedel N, Warnecke H, Adt M. Mechanical circulatory support and heart transplantation. *J Heart Lung Transplant* 1992;**11**(4 Pt 2):S175-81.
87. Loebe M, Weng Y, Muller J, et al. Successful mechanical circulatory support for more than two years with a left ventricular assist device in a patient with dilated cardiomyopathy. *J Heart Lung Transplant* 1997;**16**(11):1176-9.
88. Muller J, Wallukat G, Weng YG, et al. Weaning from mechanical cardiac support in patients with idiopathic dilated cardiomyopathy. *Circulation* 1997;**96**(2):542-9.

89. Muller J, Wallukat G, Weng YG, et al. [Temporary mechanical left heart support. Recovery of heart function in patients with end-stage idiopathic dilated cardiomyopathy]. *Herz* 1997;**22**(5):227-36.
90. Hetzer R, Muller J, Weng Y, Wallukat G, Spiegelsberger S, Loebe M. Cardiac recovery in dilated cardiomyopathy by unloading with a left ventricular assist device. *Ann Thorac Surg* 1999;**68**(2):742-9.
91. Hetzer R, Muller JH, Weng Y, Meyer R, Dandel M. Bridging-to-recovery. *Ann Thorac Surg* 2001;**71**(3 Suppl):S109-13; discussion S114-5.
92. Kumpati GS, McCarthy PM, Hoercher KJ. Left ventricular assist device as a bridge to recovery: present status. *J Card Surg* 2001;**16**(4):294-301.
93. Xydas S, Rosen RS, Ng C, et al. Mechanical unloading leads to echocardiographic, electrocardiographic, neurohormonal, and histologic recovery. *J Heart Lung Transplant* 2006;**25**(1):7-15.
94. Klotz S, Stypmann J, Welp H, et al. Does continuous flow left ventricular assist device technology have a positive impact on outcome pretransplant and posttransplant? *Ann Thorac Surg* 2006;**82**(5):1774-8.
95. Antretter H HH, Höfer D, Laufer G, Margreiter J. Totaler und partieller Herzersatz - Trends und Entwicklungen. *Journal für Kardiologie* 2002;**9**:3-13.
96. Lietz K, Miller LW. Improved survival of patients with end-stage heart failure listed for heart transplantation: analysis of organ procurement and transplantation network/U.S. United Network of Organ Sharing data, 1990 to 2005. *J Am Coll Cardiol* 2007;**50**(13):1282-90.
97. Dembitsky WP, Tector AJ, Park S, et al. Left ventricular assist device performance with long-term circulatory support: lessons from the REMATCH trial. *Ann Thorac Surg* 2004;**78**(6):2123-9; discussion 2129-30.
98. Lietz K, Miller LW. Will left-ventricular assist device therapy replace heart transplantation in the foreseeable future? *Curr Opin Cardiol* 2005;**20**(2):132-7.
99. Levin HR, Weisfeldt ML. Deep thoughts on tin men. Fact, fallacy, and future of mechanical circulatory support. *Circulation* 1997;**95**(10):2340-3.
100. Smedira NG, Blackstone EH. Postcardiotomy mechanical support: risk factors and outcomes. *Ann Thorac Surg* 2001;**71**(3 Suppl):S60-6; discussion S82-5.

101. Oz MC, Argenziano M, Catanese KA, et al. Bridge experience with long-term implantable left ventricular assist devices. Are they an alternative to transplantation? *Circulation* 1997;**95**(7):1844-52.
102. Zimpfer D, Zrunek P, Roethy W, et al. Left ventricular assist devices decrease fixed pulmonary hypertension in cardiac transplant candidates. *J Thorac Cardiovasc Surg* 2007;**133**(3):689-95.
103. Zimpfer D, Zrunek P, Sandner S, et al. Post-transplant survival after lowering fixed pulmonary hypertension using left ventricular assist devices. *Eur J Cardiothorac Surg* 2007;**31**(4):698-702.
104. Piccione W, Jr. Left ventricular assist device implantation: short and long-term surgical complications. *J Heart Lung Transplant* 2000;**19**(8 Suppl):S89-94.
105. Schmid C, Weyand M, Nabavi DG, et al. Cerebral and systemic embolization during left ventricular support with the Novacor N100 device. *Ann Thorac Surg* 1998;**65**(6):1703-10.
106. Schmid C, Weyand M, Hammel D, Deng MC, Nabavi D, Scheld HH. Effect of platelet inhibitors on thromboembolism after mplantation of a Novacor N100--preliminary results. *Thorac Cardiovasc Surg* 1998;**46**(5):260-2.
107. Arrecubieta C, Asai T, Bayern M, et al. The role of Staphylococcus aureus adhesins in the pathogenesis of ventricular assist device-related infections. *J Infect Dis* 2006;**193**(8):1109-19.
108. Vollkron M, Schima H, Huber L, Benkowski R, Morello G, Wieselthaler G. Development of a suction detection system for axial blood pumps. *Artif Organs* 2004;**28**(8):709-16.
109. Vollkron M, Schima H, Huber L, Benkowski R, Morello G, Wieselthaler G. Advanced suction detection for an axial fow pump. *Artif Organs* 2006;**30**(9):665-70.
110. Kormos RL, Borovetz HS, Gasior T, et al. Experience with univentricular support in mortally ill cardiac transplant candidates. *Ann Thorac Surg* 1990;**49**(2):261-71; discussion 271-2.
111. Kormos RL, Borovetz HS, Pristas JM, et al. LVAS pump performance following initiation of left ventricular assistance. *ASAIO Trans* 1990;**36**(3):M703-5.

112. McCarthy PM, James KB, Savage RM, et al. Implantable left ventricular assist device. Approaching an alternative for end-stage heart failure. Implantable LVAD Study Group. *Circulation* 1994;**90**(5 Pt 2):II83-6.
113. Nakatani S, Thomas JD, Savage RM, Vargo RL, Smedira NG, McCarthy PM. Prediction of right ventricular dysfunction after left ventricular assist device implantation. *Circulation* 1996;**94**(9 Suppl):II216-21.
114. Chen JM, Naka Y, Rose EA. The future of left ventricular assist device therapy in adults. *Nat Clin Pract Cardiovasc Med* 2006;**3**(7):346-7.
115. Siepe M, Heilmann C, von Samson P, Menasche P, Beyersdorf F. Stem cell research and cell transplantation for myocardial regeneration. *Eur J Cardiothorac Surg* 2005;**28**(2):318-24.
116. Potapov EV, Loebe M, Nasseri BA, et al. Pulsatile flow in patients with a novel nonpulsatile implantable ventricular assist device. *Circulation* 2000;**102**(19 Suppl 3):III183-7.
117. Frazier OH, Myers TJ, Westaby S, Gregoric ID. Use of the Jarvik 2000 left ventricular assist system as a bridge to heart transplantation or as destination therapy for patients with chronic heart failure. *Ann Surg* 2003;**237**(5):631-6; discussion 636-7.
118. Kawahito S, Takano T, Nakata K, et al. Analysis of the arterial blood pressure waveform during left ventricular nonpulsatile assistance in animal models. *Artif Organs* 2000;**24**(10):816-20.
119. Undar A, Fraser CD. Quantification of arterial pressure and pump-flow waveforms for pulsatile- and continuous-flow devices during chronic support. *J Heart Lung Transplant* 2003;**22**(6):706; author reply 706-7.
120. Prosi M, Perktold K, Schima H. Effect of continuous arterial blood flow in patients with rotary cardiac assist device on the washout of a stenosis wake in the carotid bifurcation: a computer simulation study. *J Biomech* 2007;**40**(10):2236-43.
121. Schima H, Lackner B, Prosi M, Perktold K. Numerical simulation of carotid hemodynamics in patients with rotary blood pump cardiac assist. *Int J Artif Organs* 2003;**26**(2):152-60.
122. Yada I, Golding LR, Harasaki H, et al. Physiopathological studies of nonpulsatile blood flow in chronic models. *Trans Am Soc Artif Intern Organs* 1983;**29**:520-5.

123. Taenaka Y, Tatsumi E, Nakamura H, et al. Physiologic reactions of awake animals to an immediate switch from a pulsatile to nonpulsatile systemic circulation. *ASAIO Trans* 1990;**36**(3):M541-4.
124. Golding LR, Jacobs G, Murakami T, et al. Chronic nonpulsatile blood flow in an alive, awake animal 34-day survival. *Trans Am Soc Artif Intern Organs* 1980;**26**:251-5.
125. Valdes F, Takatani S, Jacobs GB, et al. Comparison of hemodynamic changes in a chronic nonpulsatile biventricular bypass (BVB) and total artificial heart (TAH). *Trans Am Soc Artif Intern Organs* 1980;**26**:455-60.
126. Stacy D. Effects of chronic hypertension and its reversal on arteries and arterioles. *Circ Res* 1989;**65**:869–879.
127. Nishimura T, Tatsumi E, Nishinaka T, Taenaka Y, Nakata M, Takano H. Prolonged nonpulsatile left heart bypass diminishes vascular contractility. *Int J Artif Organs* 1999;**22**(7):492-8.
128. Amir O, Radovancevic B, Delgado RM, 3rd, et al. Peripheral vascular reactivity in patients with pulsatile vs axial flow left ventricular assist device support. *J Heart Lung Transplant* 2006;**25**(4):391-4.
129. Bellotto F, Johnson RG, Watanabe J, Levine MJ, Franklin A, Weintraub RM. Mechanical assistance of the left ventricle: acute effect on cardiac performance and coronary flow of different perfusion patterns. *J Thorac Cardiovasc Surg* 1992;**104**(3):561-8.
130. Losert U, Mohl W, Gogar D, et al. Regional myocardial blood flow with a nonpulsatile pump. *Int J Artif Organs* 1982;**5**(3):169-71.
131. Yozu R, Golding LA, Jacobs G, Harasaki H, Nose Y. Experimental results and future prospects for a nonpulsatile cardiac prosthesis. *World J Surg* 1985;**9**(1):116-27.
132. Tatsumi E, Toda K, Taenaka Y, et al. Acute phase responses of vasoactive hormones to non pulsatile systemic circulation. *Asaio J* 1995;**41**(3):M460-5.
133. Nishinaka T, Tatsumi E, Nishimura T, et al. Effects of reduced pulse pressure to the cerebral metabolism during prolonged nonpulsatile left heart bypass. *Artif Organs* 2000;**24**(8):676-9.
134. Moscato F, Vollkron M, Bergmeister H, Wieselthaler G, Leonard E, Schima H. Left ventricular pressure-volume loop analysis during continuous cardiac assist in acute animal trials. *Artif Organs* 2007;**31**(5):369-76.

135. Vollkron M, Voitl P, Ta J, Wieselthaler G, Schima H. Suction events during left ventricular support and ventricular arrhythmias. *J Heart Lung Transplant* 2007;**26**(8):819-25.
136. Swynghedauw B. Molecular mechanisms of myocardial remodeling. *Physiol Rev* 1999;**79**(1):215-62.
137. Birks EJ, Tansley PD, Hardy J, et al. Left ventricular assist device and drug therapy for the reversal of heart failure. *N Engl J Med* 2006;**355**(18):1873-84.
138. Haft J, Armstrong W, Dyke DB, et al. Hemodynamic and exercise performance with pulsatile and continuous-flow left ventricular assist devices. *Circulation* 2007;**116**(11 Suppl):I8-15.
139. Kashiwazaki S. Effects of artificial circulation by pulsatile and non-pulsatile flow on brain tissues. *Ann Thorac Cardiovasc Surg* 2000;**6**(6):389-96.
140. Murkin JM, Farrar JK, Tweed WA, McKenzie FN, Guiraudon G. Cerebral autoregulation and flow/metabolism coupling during cardiopulmonary bypass: the influence of PaCO2. *Anesth Analg* 1987;**66**(9):825-32.
141. Watanabe T, Miura M, Orita H, Kobayasi M, Washio M. Brain tissue pH, oxygen tension, and carbon dioxide tension in profoundly hypothermic cardiopulmonary bypass. Pulsatile assistance for circulatory arrest, low-flow perfusion, and moderate-flow perfusion. *J Thorac Cardiovasc Surg* 1990;**100**(2):274-80.
142. Anstadt MP, Tedder M, Hegde SS, et al. Pulsatile versus nonpulsatile reperfusion improves cerebral blood flow after cardiac arrest. *Ann Thorac Surg* 1993;**56**(3):453-61.
143. Zimpfer D, Wieselthaler G, Czerny M, et al. Neurocognitive function in patients with ventricular assist devices: a comparison of pulsatile and continuous blood flow devices. *Asaio J* 2006;**52**(1):24-7.
144. Polska E, Schima H, Wieselthaler G, Schmetterer L. Choroidal microcirculation in patients with rotary cardiac assist device. *J Heart Lung Transplant* 2007;**26**(6):572-8.
145. Toda K, Tatsumi E, Taenaka Y, et al. How does the sympathetic nervous system behave during non pulsatile circulation? *Asaio J* 1995;**41**(3):M465-8.
146. Henze T, Stephan H, Sonntag H. Cerebral dysfunction following extracorporeal circulation for aortocoronary bypass surgery: no differences

in neuropsychological outcome after pulsatile versus nonpulsatile flow. *Thorac Cardiovasc Surg* 1990;**38**(2):65-8.
147. Tominaga R, Smith W, Massiello A, Harasaki H, Golding LA. Chronic nonpulsatile blood flow. III. Effects of pump flow rate on oxygen transport and utilization in chronic nonpulsatile bivertricular bypass. *J Thorac Cardiovasc Surg* 1996;**111**(4):863-72.
148. Tominaga R, Smith W, Massiello A, Harasaki H, Golding LA. Chronic nonpulsatile blood flow. II. Hemodynamic responses to progressive exercise in calves with chronic nonpulsatile biventricular bypass. *J Thorac Cardiovasc Surg* 1996;**111**(4):857-62.
149. Tominaga R, Smith WA, Massiello A, Harasaki H, Golding LA. Chronic nonpulsatile blood flow. I. Cerebral autoregulation in chronic nonpulsatile biventricular bypass: carotid blood flow response to hypercapnia. *J Thorac Cardiovasc Surg* 1994;**108**(5):907-12.
150. Gaer JA, Shaw AD, Wild R, et al. Effect of cardiopulmonary bypass on gastrointestinal perfusion and function. *Ann Thorac Surg* 1994;**57**(2):371-5.
151. Wright JR, Shurrab AE, Cheung C, et al. A prospective study of the determinants of renal functional outcome and mortality in atherosclerotic renovascular disease. *Am J Kidney Dis* 2002;**39**(6):1153-61.
152. Sezai A, Shiono M, Orime Y, et al. Comparison studies of major organ microcirculations under pulsatile- and nonpulsatile-assisted circulations. *Artif Organs* 1996;**20**(2):139-42.
153. Nakata K, Shiono M, Orime Y, et al. Effect of pulsatile and nonpulsatile assist on heart and kidney microcirculation with cardiogenic shock. *Artif Organs* 1996;**20**(6):681-4.
154. Lonn U, Peterzen B, Granfeldt H, Babic A, Casimir-Ahn H. Hemopump treatment in patients with postcardiotomy heart failure. *Ann Thorac Surg* 1995;**60**(4):1067-71
155. Konishi H, Yland MJ, Brown M, et al. Effect of pulsatility and hemodynamic power on recovery of renal function. *Asaio J* 1995;**42**(5):M720-3.
156. Ohnishi H, Itoh T, Nishinaka T, et al. Morphological changes of the arterial systems in the kidney under prolonged continuous flow left heart bypass. *Artif Organs* 2002;**26**(11):974-9.

157. Maarek JM, Chartrand DA, Ye TH, Chang HK. Pulmonary lobar vascular resistances during constant and pulsatile flows. *Respir Physiol* 1990;**82**(2):149-59.
158. Johnson EH, Bennett SH, Goetzman BW. The influence of pulsatile perfusion on the vascular properties of the newborn lamb lung. *Pediatr Res* 1992;**31**(4 Pt 1):349-53.
159. Sakaki M, Taenaka Y, Tatsumi E, Nakatani T, Takano H. Influences of nonpulsatile pulmonary flow on pulmonary function. Evaluation in a chronic animal model. *J Thorac Cardiovasc Surg* 1994;**108**(3):495-502.
160. Konishi H, Sohara Y, Endo S, Misawa Y, Fuse K. Pulmonary microcirculation during pulsatile and non pulsatile perfusion. *Asaio J* 1997;**43**(5):M657-9.
161. Wieselthaler GM, Schima H, Dworschak M, et al. First experiences with outpatient care of patients with implanted axial flow pumps. *Artif Organs* 2001;**25**(5):331-5.
162. Siegenthaler MP, Martin J, Pernice K, et al. The Jarvik 2000 is associated with less infections than the HeartMate left ventricular assist device. *Eur J Cardiothorac Surg* 2003;**23**(5):748-54; discussion 754-5.
163. Hauge A, Nicolaysen G. Pulmonary O2 transfer during pulsatile and non-pulsatile perfusion. *Acta Physiol Scand* 1980;**109**(3):325-32.
164. Boldt J, Zickmann B, Dapper F, Hempelmann G. Does the technique of cardiopulmonary bypass affect lung water content? *Eur J Cardiothorac Surg* 1991;**5**(1):22-6.
165. Wieselthaler GM, Riedl M, Schima H, et al. Endocrine function is not impaired in patients with a continuous MicroMed-DeBakey axial flow pump. *J Thorac Cardiovasc Surg* 2007;**133**(1):2-6.
166. Vitali E, Lanfranconi M, Bruschi G, Russo C, Colombo T, Ribera E. Left ventricular assist devices as bridge to heart transplantation: The Niguarda Experience. *J Card Surg* 2003;**18**(2):107-13.
167. Garatti A, Bruschi G, Colombo T, et al. Clinical outcome and bridge to transplant rate of left ventricular assist device recipient patients: comparison between continuous-flow and pulsatile-flow devices. *Eur J Cardiothorac Surg* 2008;**34**(2):275-80.
168. George RS, Yacoub MH, Bowles CT, et al. Quality of life after removal of left ventricular assist device for myocardial recovery. *J Heart Lung Transplant* 2008;**27**(2):165-72.

169. Esmore DS, Kaye D, Salamonsen R, et al. Initial clinical experience with the VentrAssist left ventricular assist device: the pilot trial. *J Heart Lung Transplant* 2008;**27**(5):479-85.
170. Pae WE, Jr., Miller CA, Matthews Y, Pierce WS. Ventricular assist devices for postcardiotomy cardiogenic shock. A combined registry experience. *J Thorac Cardiovasc Surg* 1992;**104**(3):541-52; discussion 552-3.
171. Goerler H, Simon A, Gohrbandt B, et al. Cardiac retransplantation: is it justified in times of critical donor organ shortage? Long-term single-center experience. *Eur J Cardiothorac Surg* 2008.
172. Franciosa JA, Wilen M, Ziesche S, Cohn JN. Survival in men with severe chronic left ventricular failure due to either coronary heart disease or idiopathic dilated cardiomyopathy. *Am J Cardiol* 1983;**51**(5):831-6.
173. Stevenson LW. Inotropic therapy for heart failure. *N Engl J Med* 1998;**339**(25):1848-50.
174. McManus RP, O'Hair DP, Beitzinger JM, et al. Patients who die awaiting heart transplantation. *J Heart Lung Transplant* 1993;**12**(2):159-71; discussion 172.
175. Jurt U, Delgado D, Melhotra K, Bishop H, Ross H. Cardiology patient pages. Heart transplant: what to expect. *Circulation* 2002;**106**(14):1750-2.
176. Hussey JC, Parameshwar J, Banner NR. Influence of blood group on mortality and waiting time before heart transplantation in the United kingdom: implications for equity of access. *J Heart Lung Transplant* 2007;**26**(1):30-3.
177. Huang R, Deng M, Rogers JG, et al. Effect of age on outcomes after left ventricular assist device placement. *Transplant Proc* 2006;**38**(5):1496-8.
178. Badano LP, Albanese MC, De Biaggio P, et al. Prevalence, clinical characteristics, quality of life, and prognosis of patients with congestive heart failure and isolated left ventricular diastolic dysfunction. *J Am Soc Echocardiogr* 2004;**17**(3):253-61.
179. Meyns B. Indications for rotary blood pumps in clinical practice. *Artif Organs* 2001;**25**(5):323-6.
180. Vandenberghe S, Segers P, Antaki JF, Meyns B, Verdonck PR. Hemodynamic modes of ventricular assist with a rotary blood pump: continuous, pulsatile, and failure. *Asaio J* 2005;**51**(6):711-8.

181. Bolno PB, Kresh JY. Physiologic and hemodynamic basis of ventricular assist devices. *Cardiol Clin* 2003;**21**(1):15-27.
182. Kihara S, Litwak KN, Nichols L, et al. Smooth muscle cell hypertrophy of renal cortex arteries with chronic continuous flow left ventricular assist. *Ann Thorac Surg* 2003;**75**(1):178-83; discussion 183.
183. Ootaki Y, Kamohara K, Akiyama M, et al. Phasic coronary blood flow pattern during a continuous flow left ventricular assist support. *Eur J Cardiothorac Surg* 2005;**28**(5):711-6.
184. Saito S, Nishinaka T, Westaby S. Hemodynamics of chronic nonpulsatile flow: implications for LVAD development. *Surg Clin North Am* 2004;**84**(1):61-74.
185. Schima H, Vollkron M, Boehm H, et al. Weaning of rotary blood pump recipients after myocardial recovery: a computer study of changes in cardiac energetics. *J Thorac Cardiovasc Surg* 2004;**127**(6):1743-50.
186. Habazettl H, Kukucka M, Weng YG, et al. Arteriolar blood flow pulsatility in a patient before and after implantation of an axial flow pump. *Ann Thorac Surg* 2006;**81**(3):1109-11.
187. Kherani AR, Oz MC. Ventricular assistance to bridge to transplantation. *Surg Clin North Am* 2004;**84**(1):75-89, viii-ix.
188. Wei K, Kaul S. The coronary microcirculation in health and disease. *Cardiol Clin* 2004;**22**(2):221-31.
189. DeBakey ME, Teitel ER. Use of the MicroMed DeBakey VAD for the treatment of end-stage heart failure. *Expert Rev Med Devices* 2005;**2**(2):137-40.
190. Wilhelm MJ, Hammel D, Schmid C, et al. Long-term support of 9 patients with the DeBakey VAD for more than 200 days. *J Thorac Cardiovasc Surg* 2005;**130**(4):1122-9.
191. Schmid C, Tjan TD, Etz C, et al. First clinical experience with the Incor left ventricular assist device. *J Heart Lung Transplant* 2005;**24**(9):1188-94.
192. Delgado R, Bergheim M. HeartMate II left ventricular assist device: a new device for advanced heart failure. *Expert Rev Med Devices* 2005;**2**(5):529-32.
193. Deng MC, Edwards LB, Hertz MI, et al. Mechanical circulatory support device database of the International Society for Heart and Lung Transplantation: third annual report--2005. *J Heart Lung Transplant* 2005;**24**(9):1182-7.

194. Vollkron M, Schima H, Huber L, Benkowski R, Morello G, Wieselthaler G. Development of a reliable automatic speed control system for rotary blood pumps. *J Heart Lung Transplant* 2005;**24**(11):1878-85.
195. Schima H, Vollkron M, Jantsch U, et al. First clinical experience with an automatic control system for rotary blood pumps during ergometry and right-heart catheterization. *J Heart Lung Transplant* 2006;**25**(2):167-73.
196. Giridharan GA, Skliar M. Physiological control of blood pumps using intrinsic pump parameters: a computer simulation study. *Artif Organs* 2006;**30**(4):301-7.
197. Robert E, de La Coussaye JE, Aya AG, et al. Mechanisms of ventricular arrhythmias induced by myocardial contusion: a high-resolution mapping study in left ventricular rabbit heart. *Anesthesiology* 2000;**92**(4):1132-43.
198. Ziv O, Dizon J, Thosani A, Naka Y, Magnano AR, Garan H. Effects of left ventricular assist device therapy on ventricular arrhythmias. *J Am Coll Cardiol* 2005;**45**(9):1428-34.
199. Wieselthaler GM, Schima H, Wolner E. Special considerations on the implantation technique for the MicroMed-DeBakey ventricular assist device axial pump. *Ann Thorac Surg* 2003;**76**(6):2109-11.
200. Watanabe T, Yamaki M, Yamauchi S, et al. Regional prolongation of ARI and altered restitution properties cause ventricular arrhythmia in heart failure. *Am J Physiol Heart Circ Physiol* 2002;**282**(1):H212-8.
201. Brembilla-Perrot B, Villemot JP, Carteaux JP, et al. Postoperative ventricular arrhythmias after cardiac surgery: immediate- and long-term significance. *Pacing Clin Electrophysiol* 2003;**26**(2 Pt 1):619-25.
202. Chung MK. Cardiac surgery: postoperative arrhythmias. *Crit Care Med* 2000;**28**(10 Suppl):N136-44.
203. Ramaswamy K, Hamdan MH. Ischemia, metabolic disturbances, and arrhythmogenesis: mechanisms and management. *Crit Care Med* 2000;**28**(10 Suppl):N151-7.
204. Okumura K, Tsuchiya T. Idiopathic left ventricular tachycardia: clinical features, mechanisms and management. *Card Electrophysiol Rev* 2002;**6**(1-2):61-7.
205. Lerman BB, Stein KM, Markowitz SM. Mechanisms of idiopathic left ventricular tachycardia. *J Cardiovasc Electrophysiol* 1997;**8**(5):571-83.

206. Bick RJ, Bagwell SH, Jones CE, et al. Fluorescence imaging microscopy of cellular markers in ischemic vs non-ischemic cardiomyopathy after left ventricular unloading. *J Heart Lung Transplant* 2005;**24**(4):454-61.
207. Grigore A, Poindexter B, Vaughn WK, et al. Alterations in alpha adrenoreceptor density and localization after mechanical left ventricular unloading with the Jarvik flowmaker left ventricular assist device. *J Heart Lung Transplant* 2005;**24**(5):609-13.
208. Boixel C, Gonzalez W, Louedec L, Hatem SN. Mechanisms of L-type Ca(2+) current downregulation in rat atrial myocytes during heart failure. *Circ Res* 2001;**89**(7):607-13.

Acknowledgement

I would like to give my special thanks to my supervisor
Univ.-Prof. DI. Dr. H. Schima from The Center for Biomedical Engineering and Physics of the Medical University of Vienna whose help, stimulating suggestions and encouragement helped me in all the time of research for and writing of this thesis. I would like to express my gratitude to him for giving me the possibility to complete this thesis, to do the necessary research work and to use departmental data.

I have furthermore to thank Michael Vollkron from The Ludwig Boltzmann-Cluster for Cardiovascular Research, Medical University of Vienna for his skilled help and technological assistance in computing all the data as well as for his invaluable help in giving detailed explanations of the technological details behind this work.

During this thesis I have collaborated with many colleagues from
The Center for Biomedical Engineering and Physics, The Department for Cardiothoracic Surgery and The Ludwig Boltzmann-Cluster for Cardiovascular Research at the Medical University of Vienna and I want to thank all who have helped me with my work.

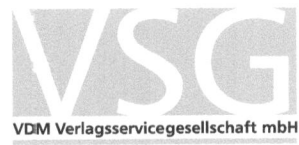

Die VDM Verlagsservicegesellschaft sucht für wissenschaftliche Verlage abgeschlossene und herausragende

Dissertationen, Habilitationen, Diplomarbeiten, Master Theses, Magisterarbeiten usw.

für die kostenlose Publikation als Fachbuch.

Sie verfügen über eine Arbeit, die hohen inhaltlichen und formalen Ansprüchen genügt, und haben Interesse an einer honorarvergüteten Publikation?

Dann senden Sie bitte erste Informationen über sich und Ihre Arbeit per Email an *info@vdm-vsg.de*.

Sie erhalten kurzfristig unser Feedback!

VDM Verlagsservicegesellschaft mbH
Dudweiler Landstr. 99
D - 66123 Saarbrücken

Telefon +49 681 3720 174
Fax   +49 681 3720 1749

www.vdm-vsg.de

Die VDM Verlagsservicegesellschaft mbH vertritt

 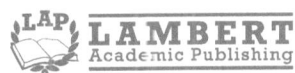 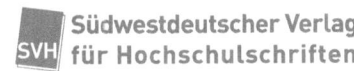

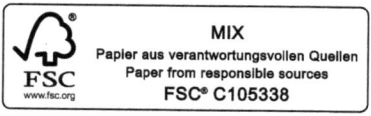

Printed by Books on Demand GmbH, Norderstedt / Germany